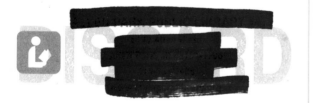

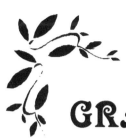
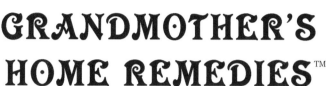

GRANDMOTHER'S
HOME REMEDIES™

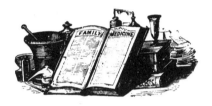

*Rediscover the secrets
Grandmothers used
to care for the
ones they loved.*

By

Dr. Myles H. Bader

Grandmother's Home Remedies™

Copyright 1997, TelAmerica Media, Inc.

All Rights Reserved

Published by: TelAmerica Media, Inc
                2044 Spruce Street
                Philadelphia, PA 19103
                (215) 732-2232

Printed in the United States of America
First printing 1997

*This book is dedicated with love to
Grandmothers everywhere
- those in body and in spirit.*

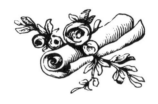

A WORD ABOUT THE AUTHOR

Dr. Myles H. Bader known by many as "Doctor Of Food Facts" has been heard on over 1200 radio and television talk shows, throughout the United States and Canada. Television appearances include: The Oprah Winfrey Show, Mike and Maty, America's Talking, The Discovery Channel (Home Matters Show), and The Morning Exchange to name just a few.

Dr. Bader received his Doctorate Degree from Loma Linda University and is board certified in Preventive Care. He has practiced in major clinics in California and is presently presenting lectures and seminars worldwide.

During the last 20 years Dr. Bader has established numerous prevention programs for Fortune 500 companies and senior organizations. These programs were in the areas of executive health, weight management, diabetes, fitness, school health and biofeedback.

Lendon Smith, M.D., better known as the Good Morning America Doctor for many years has this to say of Dr. Bader, "He is highly knowledgeable in the areas of health, nutrition and preventive medicine."

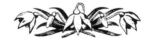

⇾ INTRODUCTION ⇽

GRANDMOTHER'S HOME REMEDIES

We've all heard the expression, "Grandmother knew best."

My Grandmother was the kind of woman that always had a pot of coffee on the stove, something wonderful smelling in the oven, and the answer for any question I could dream up. Nothing threw Grandma. "I've lived through some tough times," she use to say to me, "It'll take more than a cough or two to keep me down. "Whenever I got sick, Grandma always had "just the thing" that would make me feel better. Like her mother and grandmother before her, my Grandma had a host of home remedies that could cure whatever ailed you. Unfortunately, these invaluable pieces of homespun advice were rarely written down.

This book is about grandmother's home remedies. Not just those used by my grandmother, but those handed down from generation to generation in families everywhere. Many of the remedies used in this book originate from Native American culture. Many may remind you of your own grandmother. Others will be new to you, but may soon become part of the legacy you pass on to your family.

My Grandmother and the women like her relied on common items that were grown in their herb garden, kept in their cupboard, or bought at the general store. Often, the closest doctors were miles away - a distance that was longer still before the invention of the automobile. So, back when Grandma was a girl, they would turn to home remedies the way we would turn to our neighborhood pharmacy. In this book you'll find tried and true natural alternatives to help many common illnesses. The remedies use everyday items, herbs and foods that are easily obtainable.

1

It's important to note that the remedies do not take the place of our physician or prescribed medication, but are provided as another source of information regarding a number of illnesses and how they were treated before modern medicine came of age. Many of the remedies have been very successful and all are without side effects when used as recommended.

As you leaf through this book, I hope that some of Grandma's spirit comes through. I also hope that you will be reminded of your own grandmother and great-grandmother who have passed on a precious oral tradition that needs to be cherished. My hope is that this book will help you to continue their legacy.

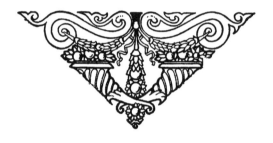

⇉ TABLE OF CONTENTS ⇇

• Contents •

• Contents •

• Contents •

• Contents •

• Contents •

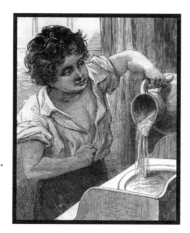

Chapter 1

TOUCHY SUBJECTS

The skin consists of three layers and is the largest organ of the body. It tends to act as a shield between the body and the thousands of foreign substances that can damage the body. Our environment contains pollutants that could harm and even kill us if they were allowed to gain entry. The skin reacts to thes harmful elements by erupting, flaking, scaling, itching, the appearance of areas of redness, color changes, cracking, and dryness.

CLEAR UP YOUR COMPLEXION: ACNE

This common skin condition occurs when the sebaceous glands, which lie just beneath the skin and produce the natural oils that keep

9

the skin lubricated, become clogged or are not regenerated in sufficient quantity to handle the load. This may result in whiteheads or
blackheads being formed. Pimples are then formed when the bacteria is released from these clogged pores.

For serious blemishes, try washing with Fels-Naptha soap, strong
stuff for oily skin. However, if your skin is normal or dry, you'll need
something gentler for your face.

Clearing Up The Outside From The Inside

Grandma, like mothers everywhere, swears that all the high-fat
food we love so much does a number on our complex-
ions. Scientists may not be quite as convinced, but to
be on the safe side, avoid chocolate, chips and fried
foods.

Eating more brown rice is good advice for improving overall
health. It is also good for your complexion. To ward off pimples and
other facial blemishes, make brown rice a regular part of your diet.

Keeping the skin and body hydrated by drinking at least eight
glasses of water daily is an effective method of keeping the skin clear
and assisting it in clearing wastes.

Studies show that zinc deficiency may contribute to acne. Be sure
to check with your doctor before taking a supplement, since too
much zinc may have harmful side-effects.

Spread It On Thick

To help fight pimples, use a paste of onion and
honey. Cook one sliced onion in a half cup honey until
it is tender. Mash with a fork to form into a paste and allow the mixture to cool. Apply to the problem area, leaving it on for an hour

before rinsing away with warm water. Use this treatment every night before going to bed until your complexion is clear and sparkling. An application of egg whites helps distribute the skin's natural oils more evenly, eliminating both dry and oily patches. Swab the egg white on your face with a cotton ball, allow to stand for five minutes and remove. Studies have shown that certain amino acids in the egg white's protein may have some anti-inflammatory properties. In most cases, small blemishes and pimples can be eliminated or reduced in size in a matter of days.

Oatmeal has long been used to control the spread of acne, as well as to speed up the healing process. Prepare the oatmeal as directed (without the milk, brown sugar, and raisins, of course!) and apply to the face. Let it stand for ten to fifteen minutes before washing off. The abrasive action of the oats cleanses deeply and increases the peripheral circulation in the affected area, which speeds up healing.

Acne and eczema as well as psoriasis have responded well to a paste made from the grain amaranth and placed on the affected area. Internally, it is taken as a tea. Take two teaspoons of the fresh seeds and cover them with boiling water, simmer on low heat for five to six minutes, remove from the heat and add two to three amaranth leaves and allow to steep for thirty to forty minutes. Two cups per day should provide relief from a number of skin problems.

Urine For A Surprise

Some folk remedies are a little strange; others are downright unappealing. I've heard that this particular cure is quite effective, so if you are really desperate about your acne you might consider trying it. Capture your first urine of the day and apply it with a washcloth to blemished skin. It works even better if you use a baby's urine, which is more pure than an adult's.

Super Strawberry Facial

If you have a chronic problem skin, try Grandma's Super Strawberry Facial. It takes a little while to prepare, so you have to plan ahead. About four hours before you'll want to go to bed, combine a cup of mashed strawberries in two cups of white cider vinegar. By the time you're ready to go to bed, it should be ready. Make sure you strain out all the solids and keep the liquid. Apply liberally to your face. Don't worry, it dries quickly. In the morning, rinse your face with warm water. It's as good an astringent as anything you can buy. Your face will feel clean and tight. It shouldn't be long before you can kiss those pimples good-bye.

Make An Astringent At Home

Blackheads respond well to lemon juice, a substance with wonderful astringent properties. Rub lemon juice over the blemished skin before going to bed and rinse with cool water in the morning. After a couple of days, you should see definite results.

Vinegar is a mild acid and cleans the affected area, reducing bacterial levels. Apply apple cider vinegar with a cotton swab and allow to stand for ten minutes before removing with a mild soap.

You'll find cucumber toners in most expensive lines of skin care products. Cucumber extract soothes skin and helps dry out acne. Juice a cucumber and apply it to your blemishes with a cotton ball. After fifteen minutes, rinse your face.

Erasing The Past

If you had a serious problem with acne in the past, you probably still have scars from it. To fade them, apply a paste consisting of one teaspoon honey mixed with a teaspoon of nutmeg. Rinse it off after twenty minutes, using cool water. Repeat this procedure twice a week. You should notice a difference within a couple of months.

Out, Out Damned Spots

In our teen years, we discovered that our grandmother had a real pet peeve about pillowcases. She blamed many common skin irritations and blemishes on dirty pillowcases, and insisted that we change them every week without fail. She reasoned that when you spend six to eight hours rubbing your face on a piece of cloth, you are bound to clear off dead skin and other residue that may contain bacteria. This idea also reinforced one of Grandma's favorite expressions: "Cleanliness is next to Godliness."

Buttermilk Facial Balm

My cousin Ruth had a terrible problem with acne as a teenager. She was very self-conscious about it. Grandma hated how unhappy it made her. "But you're such a pretty girl, Ruthie," she would always say. She started asking around among her friends and neighbors for a sure-fire cure. It was Miss Betsy, the lady next door, who came up with just the thing. Here's the recipe she shared with Grandma: Pour out a third of a cup of buttermilk and bring it to a boil. Take it off the stove and immediately start adding honey. Keep adding the honey to make up a paste, thick enough to stay where you put it. Once it's cooled, dab it on the problem areas with your fingers and leave it there for fifteen minutes before rinsing off. Cousin Ruth started using it, and before we knew it, the pimples and blackheads were completely gone.

STOP HIDING THOSE HANDS: AGE SPOTS

Age spots are areas of increased pigmentation in the skin, caused either by aging or excessive sunlight exposure. They are generally harmless. However, if they change color or cause discomfort, you should consult a physician immediately. As Grandma use to say: "An ounce of prevention is worth a pound of cure." Take care of your skin by using a sunscreen with an SPF factor of at least fifteen when going outside. Aloe vera preparations can slow down the appearance of these spots as you age.

Taking a zinc supplement may help fade age spots. However, consult your physician before trying this remedy, since high doses of zinc may have harmful side-effects.

Rub It In To Rub Them Out

Mix onion juice with twice the amount of vinegar and rub into the age spots twice a day. The brown patches should disappear before your very eyes.

Vitamin E oil is highly beneficial to the skin. It can promote healing of cuts, prevent or fade scars, and relieve dry skin. It also appears to help fade age spots. Before you go to bed, rub some Vitamin E oil into the brown patches and let it work overnight. You should see a noticeable difference in a few weeks.

• *Skin Solutions* •

Lemon juice can be used as a temporary measure to bleach out age spots. Dab a small amount on the spot and allow it to dry. For the best results, this should be repeated at least two to three times each day. It may take two to three months before you see results.

Give It Some Time

Apply buttermilk compresses to the area for twenty minutes twice each day. The mild lactic acid found in milk products appears to be the active ingredient. Due to individual differences in skin, treatment time may vary.

The herb gota kola has been used for hundreds of years for memory problems. It also works on age spots. Mix a solution of a quarter teaspoon powdered gota kola, a half cup very hot water and an eighth teaspoon Korean ginseng. Place a poultice on the areas and let stand ten minutes. Apply twice a day. You should see results in about one month. Gota kola is an effective bleaching agent, but it may take longer than some of the other treatments.

Fountain Of Youth Food

Chick peas are a veritable fountain of youth. They are low in fat, high in fiber and nutrients, all of which will keep you feeling youthful and energetic. You can also use them to fade age spots. You can buy them dried or canned. If dried, prepare them according to the directions on the package. Mash up a small bowl of them and add enough water to make a paste. Rub the chickpeas over the brown places, letting it stay until it dries, and then wash your hands. If you keep doing this every day, your hands will start looking years younger.

LEAVE IT IN THE LOCKER ROOM: ATHLETE'S FOOT

Athlete's foot is a fungal infection that thrives in dark, warm locations. It is very contagious, and you should not walk barefoot on a gym or locker room floor.

When she could get to the store, Grandma picked up some over-the-counter antifungal remedies to have on hand for whoever needed them. Try Desenex or Tinactin. The question of cream versus powder is really one of personal preference. Some people like the crisp, dryness of powders, while others enjoy a cream's moisturizing effect.

Rubbing your feet to remove dead skin cells may help relieve the problem and prevent the fungus from spreading.

Grandma's Secret Foot Soak

One of Grandma's favorite recipes for athletes foot: Mix together a half cup chlorine bleach, a quarter cup apple cider vinegar, and two tablespoons of salt in one gallon of warm water. Soak your feet for twenty minutes twice a day until the problem goes away.

Smelly Solutions

Garlic can destroy foot fungus. Dust feet with garlic powder, not garlic salt, before putting on your socks.

Another effective way to kill the fungus is to soak your feet in a vinegar bath. Mix a half cup apple cider vinegar in one gallon of warm filtered water for at least ten to fifteen minutes twice a day. Allow your feet to air dry afterwards.

16

Gooey But Good for You

Other effective natural treatments include: applying tea tree oil directly to the site, diluting fifteen drops of eucalyptus oil in one tablespoon olive oil and applying the solution two times per day.

Soak some cloth with honey and tape it to the bottoms of your feet. You'll want to wear socks over the top of it to keep the mess from getting everywhere. Wear this honey poultice to bed. In the morning, undo it and wash your feet, drying thoroughly and applying some powder or cornstarch to keep them dry. Your athlete's foot should clear up quickly.

Break off a piece of your aloe vera plant to cure athlete's foot. Rub the gel into your feet two times a day, in the morning and in the evening. If you don't have a green thumb, you can also buy aloe vera gel or juice at the local health food store. Even stubborn athlete's foot has been known to respond to this treatment.

Beachy Keen

Everything is better at the beach, including your athlete's foot problem. Salt seems to kill the fungus that causes the itching. If you don't live close enough to the ocean for frequent strolls, soak your feet for five to ten minutes a day in a pint of warm water with two teaspoons salt dissolved in it. Continue until the problem clears up.

The Dry Idea

Keeping your feet dry helps keep athlete's foot away. Pay careful attention to your feet and in-between toes after you shower. If toweling doesn't seem enough, use your blow-dryer. Cornstarch or baking soda can help keep feet dry.

My grandmother was a practical woman. It made sense to her that if an anti-perspirant could keep your underarms dry it could do the same for your feet. Try your roll-on or spray to combat athlete's foot.

Some people didn't believe Grandma when she told them to wear white socks to get rid of athlete's foot, but white socks are free from dyes that may aggravate skin problems. Choose socks made from absorbent, natural fibers to avoid foot fungus.

Aloha To Foot Fungus

You'll think you're in the islands when you use Grandma's pineapple footbath to rid your feet of fungus. You'll need to plan for this remedy, since you need to leave your feet in pineapple juice for an hour. When the calypso music ends and the hour is up, dry your feet and sprinkle with baking soda. If you repeat this every day, your athlete's foot problem should clear up quickly.

Keep Your Socks On

A foot soak is very relaxing, but if you add astringent ingredients, such as Epsom salts, lemon juice, vinegar, black tea, chlorine beach, or borax, it will help kill bacteria and reduce sweating which will stop foot odor. Mix a quarter cup white vinegar and two to three tablespoon of Epsom salts in a half gallon of water for an effective, germ-fighting foot soak.

Once again, baking soda comes to the rescue. Sprinkle it on your feet to absorb odor. Place a small amount in your shoes or socks.

TAKE OFF THE PRESSURE: BED SORES

These ulcerated areas form when too much pressure is exerted over a bony area. This causes a restriction of circulation, resulting in the death of cells and the overlying tissue. The most common area for bedsores is the base of the spine caused by lying in bed for prolonged periods. Massage the area to improve circulation and change positions regularly to prevent sores.

Eat one cup spinach each day for a week. Garlic also helps speed healing.

SORE SPOTS: BOILS

Boils, also called furuncle, are round, pus-filled, reddened and raised areas on the skin. They are usually caused by an infected wound, poor hygiene, a food allergy or stress.

Kitchen Cures

Apply honey directly to the boil. Another method is to use very warm clay packs four to five times a day if possible. Also an onion poultice can be used between a piece of cloth but not placed directly on the boil.

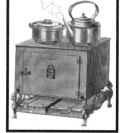

You can also use pumpkin, lemon, and figs to bring a boil to a head. Apply slices of fresh pumpkin to the boil, replacing them until the boil is better. Warm up a lemon in the oven, cut in half, and apply to the boil, securing it in place. Leave it on the boil for an hour. In the Bible, the prophet Isaiah suggests figs to cure a boil. In your oven, roast a fresh fig, cut it in half, remove the flesh, and place it on the boil. Keep it in place with a bandage or cloth, for a couple of before the boil is gone.

Grandma knew as much about baking as she did about home cures. When somebody got a boil, she used both these skills, making a poultice of bread and milk. You don't have to use homemade bread, but my grandmother would recommend it.

Try oatmeal on a boil, as a warm poultice, kept in place with a bandage. Leave overnight.

Slices of raw potato or cooked onion may also help bring a boil to a head.

Grandmother's Egg-cellent Boil Cure

Grandmother had a very unusual method for eliminating painful boils. She would boil an egg and remove the lining, the small thin membrane layer that lies just under the shell, and place it on the boil covered with a band-aid. In most cases, this will bring the boil to a head by morning. Important note: Make sure the egg has been boiled for at least fifteen minutes before removing the membrane because salmonella contamination is always possible and placing any part of a raw egg near an open wound may be cause for concern. Eggs, even if unbroken when purchased, may be contaminated with bacteria.

Boil Brews

A milk-based poultice will help bring a boil to a head. Gently heat one cup milk, add three teaspoons of salt gradually as the milk nears the boiling point. Remove from the stove and add flour to the mixture until it forms a paste. Apply to the affected area, making sure that it is not so hot that it will burn the skin. In a few days, the boil will break, releasing pus, and the pain will be gone.

· Skin Solutions ·

If you have a boil, brew yourself a cup of tea, enjoy, and put the still-warm tea bag on the boil. The warmth helps draw out the toxins, and acids in the tea may kill some kinds of bacteria.

Take a small bottle, fill with warm water, not too hot, and carefully put on top of the boil. The suction action will draw out pus.

Fat Will Do The Trick

Beef fat is bad for your arteries but good for a boil. Melt some fat and add to a small amount of pine sap. Apply to the boil.

Bacon fat can also help rupture a boil. Place it on the affected area and attach with a gauze dressing or Band-Aid. Keep changing the bacon fat to keep it fresh until the boil is better.

Another of Grandma's favorite remedies was to use a small amount of coal tar under a Band-Aid overnight. This has an excellent drawing affect, but is a bit messy. Be careful since it will contaminate an open wound.

A "Fishy" Boil Cure

When you're a kid, you don't care if something is good for you. If it tastes bad, you want to steer as far away from it as possible. Grandma used cod liver oil to treat a number of ailments, and I tried to avoid each and every one of them. At least with a boil, the cod liver oil went on the outside, not down the throat. To make your own "Fishy" Boil Cure, combine a tablespoon of cod liver oil with a tablespoon of honey. Put a handful on the boil and bandage it up. Make sure you change the bandage regularly, at least every eight hours.

THE BLACK AND BLUE BLUES: BRUISES

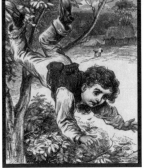

Bruising occurs when the skin is not broken, but the underlying tissues are injured. This results in small blood vessels being broken, causing localized pain, swelling, and a black-and-blue area.

Tea And C

Drink twelve ounces of orange juice a day. Vitamin C strengthens the walls of the blood vessels. Taking a Vitamin C supplement of 500-1,000 milligrams a day will also work wonders for repeated bruising.

Severe bruises involving broken blood vessels and skin discoloration respond well to the herb ledum. Take as a tea or apply externally to the affected area.

Fade Away

Apply an icepack to a bruise or immerse the affected area in cold water to reduce swelling and fade black-and-blue marks more quickly. Do not place ice directly on skin or use water that is painfully cold. This remedy is effective because it constricts blood vessels and there is less bleeding beneath the skin.

Gently apply witch hazel to the bruised area to speed up healing and help the mark fade. Witch hazel also constricts blood vessels to lessen bleeding. Natural witch hazel may be more effective than commercial preparations. Boil one teaspoon powdered leaves or twigs in a cup of water, strain, and cool. Apply the ointment to the bruised area.

Don't Knock It Til You Try It

Apply a poultice of grated turnip to a bruise to promote faster healing. Leave it in place for up to half an hour.

Boil a small amount of comfrey leaves for ten minutes, and let cool. Soak the bruised area in the mixture or apply as a poultice.

Carefully apply a salve of parsley and a teaspoon of butter to a bruise. It should soothe the sore area and help fade the black-and-blue mark.

Keep It From Coloring

To prevent a bruised area from discoloring, try any of these three remedies. Right after you bump into the end table or knock your leg against the car door, head for your kitchen and break out the sugar. With moistened fingers, gently rub the sugar across the injured area. The next day, you should wake up without any trace of black or blue. You can also prevent a bruise by applying an arrowroot paste, a couple of tablespoons of arrowroot and a little water, to the skin. It will dry up and fall off, leaving behind unblemished skin. When you get a bruise, eat a banana and rub the skin with the inside of the peel. To completely ward off a bruise, secure the peel to the injured area and leave overnight. By morning, there should be no bruise to speak of.

Don't-Drink-Me Tea

Try this Italian cure for a nasty bruise that helps relieve pain and swelling. Brew a tea from one large tablespoon of oregano and a cup of boiling water. Let it set for ten minutes and strain. Put the wet oregano in a piece of cloth and apply to the bruise. Keep the liquid to refresh the oregano leaves.

How To Sweeten Up A Bruise

Grandma kept a huge jar of blackstrap molasses in her kitchen, but it wasn't with her baking supplies. She kept it in the cupboard with the other ingredients for her home remedies. Whenever I'd come home from school all black and blue from horsing around, she'd tear off a piece of brown paper and dip it in the molasses. She'd secure it to the bruise with a bandage, and several hours later when she took it off, the bruise would be almost completely gone.

TOO CLOSE TO THE FLAME: BURNS

There are three different degrees of burns. First degree burns, the least serious, are identified by redness only, second degree by redness and blistering, and the most serious, third degree burns by the destruction of the skin and underlying muscle. Third degree burns need a physician's care as soon as possible to avoid serious infection.

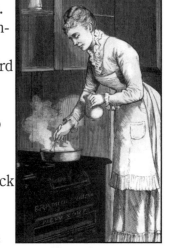

If Grandma could get to the store, she'd pick up some over-the-counter remedies that helped relieve the pain of burns. Many of these commercial preparations contain active ingredients to deaden pain, as well as ingredients to fight infection. Many also contain aloe vera which is soothing to burned skin.

Sweet Relief

Sometimes when my grandmother was baking, she would burn herself taking a pie out of the oven. Whenever that happened, she'd take a small piece of pie crust dough rolled thin and put in on the burn, leaving it until it dried up. By the time it fell off, the pain from the burn would be completely gone.

• *Skin Solutions* •

For a sweet burn cure, apply honey to the affected area to ease pain. Since bacteria will not grow on honey, it also promotes quick healing and prevents infection. Some people feel that the honey is more effective if combined with sauerkraut or comfrey root.

Layers of apple butter can help heal a burn. Spread apple butter over the affected area and keep reapplying as each coat dries. Keep this up for a day or two, and the burn should be well on its way to healing.

Swell Advice

Place a cold compress on the affected area to reduce swelling and pain. The burned area should be elevated to reduce swelling.

Quick Relief

Apply aloe vera to first degree burns immediately, and to second and third degree burns after healing has begun.

If you're outside and need an immediate treatment for a burn, apply mud to the area to cool the skin.

A burned tongue can really hurt. For a severe problem, wash your mouth out with cool water until it starts to feel better. You may also want to try a few drops of vanilla extract to ease the pain.

When burned by hot wax, tar, or melted plastic, use ice water to harden the material before trying to remove it.

Don't Eat Your Vegetables

Apply layers of sliced raw potatoes to the burn, refreshing every few minutes. The starch in the potatoes will form a protective coating of starch to soothe the skin. You can also use a piece of fresh pumpkin or onion.

• Skin Solutions •

You can use items out of the refrigerator, mushrooms and radishes, to soothe a burn. Slice a mushroom and put the pieces on your burned skin to promote healing. You can use the radishes to make a poultice for the burn. Make sure that they are cold, straight out of the refrigerator. Puree in a blender and apply to the burn.

The Carrot Juice Cure

Grandma had an unusual treatment for a burn or a scald. She would immediately soak the affected area in ice water and then place a dressing dipped in pure carrot juice on the area. She repeated this three to four times a day for about three days.

Grandma's Open Cupboard Cures

Try the vinegar and brown paper bag cure for a burn. Soak a piece of brown bag in white cider vinegar. Placing it on the affected area should have a cooling effect and relieve the pain.

Applying baking soda mixed with extra virgin olive oil to first and second degree burns will promote healing and reduce the chances of scarring.

Vitamin E oil helps skin heal more quickly and prevents scarring and blistering. Apply liberally to the area several times a day and bandage with sterile gauze. This vitamin's anti-oxidant properties may help reduce inflammation.

Vanilla extract relieves the pain of a grease burn.

Place a piece of charcoal on a burn and leave it for at least an hour. The pain will quickly subside. When you take away the charcoal, much of the redness should have disappeared.

Comfort From Within

Once a burn has started to heal, make a strong tea from blackberry leaves and apply on a compress two to three times a day to speed healing.

To relieve the discomfort of second and third degree burns, increase the low-fat protein in your diet to at least 3,000-4,000 calories a day. Drink at least eight to ten glasses of water a day.

SMOOTHING THE ROUGH SPOTS: CORNS AND CALLUSES

Calluses are formed when the body tries to protect itself from a severe irritation by building up excess hard protective tissues that are usually flat. Corns are formed as a result of pressure which forces the body to build up raised layers of skin, causing pain.

You're Soaking In It

Give your feet a soothing bath in oatmeal water. Add a little less than two cups of oats to five quarts boiling water. Boil down to four quarts of liquid, remove from heat, and strain, retaining the liquid. Soak your feet for twenty minutes or more.

A good warm soak, plain water or with a variety of ingredients, will help tired feet feel better and can reduce discomfort from corns and calluses. Try adding a little vinegar, iodine, Epsom salts, or baking soda to the water for added effectiveness.

Stop It Before It Starts

Grandma preferred to prevent a problem whenever she could. She

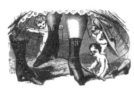

didn't have much patience with fancy shoes that didn't fit right and caused foot problems. Comfort, comfort, comfort, that was her motto. She particularly recommended avoiding high heels and shoes with pointy toes.

Callus And Corn Coverage

Dissolve six crushed aspirin in one tablespoon of water. Apply to the corn or callous to treat it. Don't use this remedy if you are allergic to aspirin.

Soak one crumbled piece of bread in a quarter cup of vinegar, letting it stand for thirty minutes. Apply to the corn as a poultice and tape in place. Leave it on overnight, and by morning, the corn should easily come off. If it doesn't, repeat the remedy several times, until the corn falls off.

Tape a piece of pineapple peel to your corn, with the flesh-side against your skin. Replace every day until the corn is gone.

There is nothing nicer than a hot cup of tea, and you can recycle the used tea bag as a remedy for your corns. After your morning cup of tea, secure the tea bag to your corn and leave for half an hour. Keep doing this every day until the corn disappears in a week or two.

Getting Ready For Bed

Every night before going to bed, rub some vitamin E oil, available at your local health food store, into the corn or callus, massaging for a couple of minutes. Let your feet air day for a few minutes before putting on a pair of socks and turning in for the night. After a couple of nights of this treatment, a corn should fall off and a callous should be softened.

Cut a small piece of lemon and secure it to the corn, pulling on a pair of socks to keep it in place overnight. Keep doing this until the corn is gone.

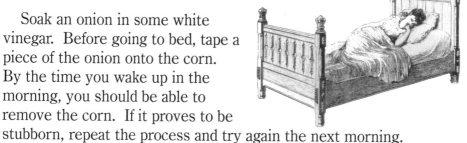

Soak an onion in some white vinegar. Before going to bed, tape a piece of the onion onto the corn. By the time you wake up in the morning, you should be able to remove the corn. If it proves to be stubborn, repeat the process and try again the next morning.

If a corn or callus is really bothering you, apply lemon juice or vinegar as a poultice and leave overnight. It will help soften the spot, so you can remove dead skin.

Grandpa's Pampered Feet

Hardworking folks like my grandmother know the importance of taking care of their feet. When Grandpa would come home from a hard day at work complaining about his "aching dogs," Grandma would just shake her head and reach for the basin. Before Grandpa could change out of his work clothes, Grandma would soak his feet in a solution of castor oil. Then she would use an emery board or pumice stone to remove the dead skin. Although he complained and moaned the whole time, we knew that Grandpa loved all the pampering.

FAREWELL TO FLAKES: DANDRUFF

Dandruff is caused by scalp glands that do not function properly, causing drying and then scaling of the skin. Itching and burning may occur in serious cases, and a physician should be consulted before any treatment at home.

In some cases, exposure to sunlight will help. Also try consuming one serving of yogurt a day for a week.

Nothing Flaky About This Cure

 Grandmother's favorite method of getting rid of dandruff was her special scalp massage. Mix one cup apple cider vinegar in one cup of water and add ten mint leaves. Bring this mixture to a boil for five minutes, then allow to stand at room temperature for twelve hours. Strain and massage into the scalp twice each day for seven days. There is no need to rinse; the mixture will dissipate and will not leave an odor.

Wash Those Flakes Right Out Of Your Hair

A shampoo of the herb bay laurel eliminates dandruff. Prepare the solution with one quart boiling water and three to four teaspoons of crushed bay laurel leaves. Allow to steep for thirty minutes, strain and allow to stand in the refrigerator for one hour. After you wash your hair with your normal shampoo, massage some of the tea into your scalp. Repeat the treatment a second time and allow it stay on your scalp for one hour before rinsing. The herbal shampoo needs to be used regularly for the best results.

A traditional Arab remedy for dandruff recommends washing the hair with a mixture of one cup beet juice, two cups water, and one teaspoon salt. If you've ever dripped beet juice on your clothes, you know that it acts as a dye. So if you have light-colored hair, don't use this remedy, unless you fancy something in a light pink.

Try a lemon rinse to banish dandruff. Apply the juice of half a large lemon to your hair, wash your hair with your regular shampoo, and rinse. Mix the other half of the juice with two cups of water, and rinse again. Continue using this lemony rinse every other day until you are without flakes.

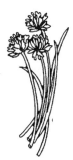

Shampoo your hair as you usually would and rinse with chive tea. To make the brew, let a tablespoon of chives steep in a cup of boiling water for twenty minutes. If you follow this treatment once a week, it should fight off your dandruff problem.

Thyme For A Cure

Grandma would brew up a batch of thyme rinse to treat dandruff. Boil four tablespoons of dried thyme, using two cups of water, for ten minutes. Strain and cool. Use half of the mixture to rinse damp hair making sure it gets to the scalp, and keep the other half for another time.

A derivative of thyme oil is an active ingredient in Lysterine. If you'd rather go to the drug store than the health food store, pick up some Lysterine and massage into the wet scalp with a cotton ball, waiting an hour or so before washing your hair. Repeating several times a week for a couple of weeks should clear up the dandruff.

A Flowery Solution

Grandma recommended washing your hair with a mixture of ginger and chamomile flowers, an ounce of each, to cure dandruff. She'd tie them up in a handkerchief and boil for ten minutes in a gallon of water. She'd let it cool and seal it tightly in a bottle to store it. Grandpa had problems with dandruff from time to time. So she'd have him wash his hair and rinse with a handful of her ginger-chamomile brew. She'd tell him not to rinse, just to leave it in, and before long, the flakes would be gone.

If Grandma didn't have time to whip up her ginger brew, she'd snip a leaf off her trusty aloe vera plant for a quick scalp soother. She'd squeeze out the gel and rub it into Grandpa's hair and scalp. Then she'd wrap his head up in a towel. The next morning Grandpa would wash his hair, without any shampoo, letting the aloe vera go to work. Grandpa's dandruff would soon be history.

Here's The Rub

Grandma always recommended that we massage our scalp to keep the skin healthy. She often turned to the items sitting on her kitchen shelf as home remedies. For dandruff, wash your hair, massage in a little warm olive oil, wrap your head with a towel, and leave overnight. In the morning, brush your hair to loosen dandruff flakes, and rinse out the oil. One of the causes of dandruff is a dry scalp, and an occasional warm oil treatment will remedy that in a jiffy. You don't want to overdo, however, since too much oil can make the problem worse.

One way to relieve your dry scalp without making your hair oily is to use this massage and soak method. Pour out enough peanut oil to massage into your entire scalp and warm it up before applying. Rinse with lemon juice and let both ingredients work for fifteen minutes before shampooing with baby shampoo. You can use corn oil in much the same way.

FLAKY, SCALY, ITCHY: DERMATITIS

Dermatitis is an allergic reaction that causes flaking, scaling and itching of the skin. Metals are frequently the cause, but creams, ointments, and certain plants may also be the culprit. Dermatitis tends to spread and may become a serious problem.

Apply a mixture of the herb goldenseal and vitamin E with a small amount of honey to add consistency. Leave on the affected area for twenty to thirty minutes and use at least three times a day.

HOW TO BE A SMOOTHIE: DRY SKIN

Nature's Healing Hand

A traditional Hawaiian remedy for dry skin is kukui nut oil. It's great for both face and body. The oil is pleasant-smelling and absorbs quickly, without a heavy, greasy feeling.

For dry skin care, try cleaning your face in whole milk. Add 1 teaspoon of castor oil to three tablespoons of warm milk. Shake well to mix and apply to your face with a cotton ball. This milk and oil mixture is terrific for removing makeup and dirt.

Dry skin may be alleviated by using a chamomile and lavender preparation.

Over-The-Counter Curatives

For chronic dry skin, try Eucerin, an over-the-counter product that contains mineral oil and lanolin, ingredients that help your skin retain moisture.

The farm hands at Grandma's stumbled on a great treatment for dry skin, Bag Balm, a product that helps soothe a mother cow who is nursing. It's especially good for the stubborn, dry skin on the bottom of the feet. Apply it thoroughly before bedtime and put on socks to keep it from getting on the sheets. You can use Vaseline in the same way, on the tough skin of elbows, knees and feet. Take a bath before bed, apply the jelly to your feet, and pull on socks.

Petroleum jelly is also an effective facial moisturizer. Glob some of the petroleum jelly on your fingertips and rub on your face and neck. Keep adding water to continually thin the layer of jelly on your face until it no longer feels greasy.

Nutrition Solution

Sulfur, found in onions, garlic, asparagus, and eggs, tends to keep the skin smooth with a youthful appearance.

Another Reason To Quit

Smoking dries out skin and causes premature wrinkling around the mouth.

PAMPER YOUR FACE FRESH: FACIAL MASKS

Facials are a wonderful idea for skin health and beauty. It's best to apply facials in the evening, when your skin will be free of makeup for several hours. Facial masks are most effective after a shower or bath, after your face has been gently steamed and the pores are open. Always start with a clean face and neck and rub the mixtures in with an upward circular motion.

The Banana Mask

This is an excellent mask for dry skin. It's also recommended to reduce and prevent fine lines and wrinkles. Mash a ripe banana with a drop or two of peanut oil. Spread it on your face and neck and leave on for about a half an hour. Remove with lukewarm water. You may apply this mask every day or every other day to promote softer skin.

The Cocoa Powder Mask

Cocoa powder may be a popular baking ingredient but it also makes one of the best masks for a dry skin problem. Prepare a mixture of two cups cocoa powder, two tablespoons dairy cream, and one to two tablespoons extra virgin olive oil. The consistency may have to be worked with and the ingredients altered slightly until you have a thick paste, one that won't fall off too easily once applied. The olive oil will prevent the mixture from drying out prematurely. The mixture is approximately twenty-five to thirty percent linoleic acid which is the ingredient that will do the job. The reason grandma's skin always looked great was this inexpensive solution. She never had the money to purchase all those fancy skin preparations.

The Eggplant Yogurt Mask

This is a fine mask for oily skin. Blend a quarter of a small eggplant with its skin and one cup of plain yogurt in a blender. Spread over your face, being careful to avoid the delicate skin around your eyes. Leave on for twenty minutes then rinse with lukewarm water. You might want to finish this treatment off with an astringent or toner. Keep chamomile tea in a spray bottle in your refrigerator and spritz the tea on your face after you rinse off the mask, or use anytime as a quick skin refresher.

The Egg White Wrinkle Mask

This mask is said to smooth the wrinkles associated with age. You can apply this mask three or four times a week. Mix an egg white with some sweet cream. Lightly spread around your eye area and let it set for half an hour to an hour. Rinse with lukewarm water.

The Honey Mask

Apply unheated honey to your face with your fingertips. Spread with an upward circular motion. Rinse with lukewarm water after twenty minutes. This sticky mask should aid in ridding your complexion of blackheads and blemishes. You'll feel refreshed.

The Honey And Cream Mask

This is another good mask that has a good reputation for helping wrinkles. Mix one teaspoon of honey with two tablespoons of heavy whipping cream. Mix very well. With your fin-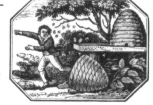gertips, gently massage the mixture into the fine lines and wrinkles on your face. Leave on for at least half an hour. You'll feel a gentle tightening. When you've had enough, rinse off with lukewarm water. I've heard that people have made this a part of their evening ritual and many swear by the results. You be the judge.

The Oatmeal Cleansing Mask

In a blender, place one cup of uncooked oatmeal and blend until it's reduced to a powder. Mix the powder with one egg white, a half cup of skim milk and three drops of almond oil. Spread the mask on your face and neck—avoiding the tender area around your eyes. Leave on for half an hour before rinsing with lukewarm water.

The Oily Oatmeal Mask

Add vegetable oil to cooked oatmeal—just enough to make it easy to spread. Massage into your face and neck. After half an hour, wash off with lukewarm water. If used daily, this mask may reduce wrin-kles.

The Papaya Mask

You'll need a blender for this one. Peel a ripe papaya and puree. Spread the pureed fruit on your face and leave on for twenty minutes. Rinse with lukewarm water. This refreshing mask will help remove dead skin cells.

The Too-Much Sun Mask

This mask is not for sunburns, rather, it's for skin that has been enduring years of sun abuse—the kind often called "leathery." Mix two tablespoons of flour into two tablespoons of raw honey. Add about three tablespoons of milk—enough to make the mixture the consistency of toothpaste. Smooth the paste on your face and neck with your fingertips, avoiding the delicate area around your eyes. Leave on for twenty minutes and rinse off with lukewarm water. Pat dry. Follow with a toner and moisturizer.

SOOTHING RELIEF: ITCHING

Chronic itching comes from rashes, skin irritations and allergic reactions.

A Dab Will Do You

The nuisance of itching can easily be controlled by using a salve made from chickweed. Place one and a half cups diced chickweed in two cups extra virgin olive oil that has been heated with five tablespoons of beeswax. Combine all ingredients and place in a 200 degree oven for two hours. Strain the mixture while it is still warm (before the wax solidifies) and place into a clean jar that can be sealed tightly.

Rubbing freshly sliced carrots on an itchy spot can give you relief. Slices of raw onion will also do the trick.

One way to prevent getting itchy, dry skin is to moisturize regularly. Especially in the winter months. For best absorption, apply the moisturizer while your skin is moist, after a bath or shower.

Taking The "Bite" Out

Mosquito bite sufferers may find welcome relief from witch hazel. Just dab it on the bite and your urge to itch will go away. The witch hazel may also help reduce swelling.

In the summertime, Grandma used to give us ice to rub on our mosquito bites. It always stopped the itching for a while, and the swelling went down, too. Taking a cool shower is another way to temporarily relieve itchy skin.

Immerse Yourself In Relief

Among its many uses, baking soda helps to relieve the itching associated with chicken pox, insect bites and other itchy afflictions. Make a paste with baking soda and water and dab it on the bite or itchy spot. You'll find it will soothe the itch and keep you from scratching—an important factor in aiding healing. You may even try pouring some in your bath. If you prefer showers, wet your skin then pour some baking soda into your hands and apply to the areas that itch. Leave on for a few minutes before rinsing. Don't make the bath or shower water too hot. The hot water will make you feel even itchier.

For those who are fortunate enough to live by the ocean, salt water does wonders for itchy skin. The salt water will not only help stop the itching, it can help to dry blisters and kill some kinds of fungus. Landlubbers can make a soak by adding two tablespoons of salt (table salt will do) to a pint of lukewarm water. Soak for five or ten minutes and repeat as needed.

Many skin ailments such as allergic reactions, eczema, poison ivy and chicken pox can be soothed by taking an oatmeal bath. Put some oatmeal in netting fine enough to keep the oats inside (even a sock or old pantyhose will do). Then place it in the bathtub (like a tea bag) while the water is filling and have a good long soak. Make sure the bath water is warm, not hot. One bath might do the trick, but repeat for a few days if necessary. You may also try a finely ground oat product called colloidal oatmeal. You can find one or more varieties at your local pharmacy. Take colloidal oatmeal baths once or twice a day.

Snacking Solutions

Here's a "snack" that can help to relieve itching. Mix a few tea-spoons of ground flaxseeds with dried fruit and nuts. Ground flaxseed or flaxseed oil can improve the itch of psoriasis. If you are taking anti-clotting agents or aspirin, check with your doctor before consuming.

Sometimes changing your diet can alleviate itching. Make sure to eat plenty of foods rich in iron. These include leafy green vegetables, fish and dried fruit. Taking iron supplements can be beneficial, too. Ask your doctor for the recommended dosage.

IN NEED OF A MANICURE: NAIL PROBLEMS

Nails can become fragile, dry, ridged, brittle or have white bands.

An Ounce Of Prevention

My Grandmother wore rubber gloves when she did the dishes, a practice that seems to have gone out of fashion. You can still buy these gloves at any store and they're terrific for protecting your hands and nails from harsh detergents and bleach. You may find that you are sensitive to rubber gloves, but don't throw them out. Simply wear vinyl gloves under the rubber ones, and you should be fine.

Nail Nutrients

Carrot juice, approximately one cup a day, should relieve dryness and brittleness. Increase intake of whole grains to strengthen nails and eliminate ridges. Hangnails and white bands are usually a sign of a low-protein diet.

If you have a problem with splitting fingernails, eat six raw almonds a day. The almonds are a good source of protein, vitamins and nutrients, plus an ingredient called linoleic acid that helps keep nails healthy. You'll have to keep this up for a while before you notice the results.

Smoothing The Rough Edges

While you're making your hands look lovely with moisturizers, don't neglect your nails. Hard, brittle nails can often be helped with hand creams. Nails that break easily may be helped by massaging in a little petroleum jelly. But be careful: soft nails will be made softer by too much moisturizing cream.

If you browse the shampoo aisle of your local store, you may 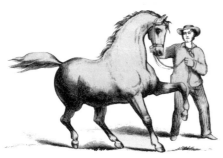 notice a few brands that claim to have been developed by horse trainers. Well, horse trainers have also developed a product that's terrific for hands and nails. Called "Hoof Saver," this is a cream used on horses by vets and animal trainers. It's great for maintaining strong, hard nails. It's inexpensive and contains many of the ingredients found in the hand creams used by humans. Try looking for Hoof Saver in feed stores.

You're Soaking In It

Here's a remedy the character Madge would love (if you remember Madge, you're dating yourself). Steep one tablespoon of horsetail in a cup of boiling water. Once it cools a bit, strain the horsetail. Then, soak your fingers in it. If you do this every day, you'll see improvement in about a month.

DULLING THE SHINE: OILY SKIN

Squeaky Clean

Oily skin may be alleviated by using a liquid made from lemon grass and licorice root.

A good cleanser for oily skin is one you can mix up at home. Take one tablespoon of powdered milk and mix in water until it takes on a milky consistency. Apply the mixture with a cotton ball, gently rubbing it into your face and neck. While it's still moist, wipe off the makeup and dirt with a tissue. Pat dry.

Toning Up

If you don't mind smelling like a pickle, this toner is terrific for restoring the pH balance of your skin. Mix one tablespoon of boiled water with one tablespoon of apple cider vinegar. As soon as it cools to a comfortable temperature, dip in a cotton ball and apply to your face. Your skin will feel smooth and tight, but be aware that the fumes from the vinegar may make your eyes a little teary.

Cucumbers have long been used as a beauty aid. Here's a cucumber toner you can make yourself. Juice two cucumbers in a juice extractor and heat the liquid until boiling, skimming off any froth that might appear. Place in a bottle or jar and keep in the refrigerator. You can use this toner twice a day, after you've washed your face. Mix one teaspoon of the cucumber juice with two tea-spoons of water. Gently apply to your face and neck. Let dry before using a moisturizer.

From The Inside Out

For oily skin, try drinking yarrow tea each day. Yarrow is a natural astringent and can cut down on the oils in your skin. Use one table-spoon of dried yarrow to one cup of boiling water. Let steep for about ten minutes. Strain before drinking.

THE NASTY SIDE OF NATURE: POISON IVY AND POISON OAK

When bare skin comes in contact with the sap of the poison ivy or oak plant, it develops redness, rash, blistering and swelling in sus-ceptible individuals. Scratching makes the problem worse and may transmit it to other parts of the body. Animals that come into contact with the plant can transmit the sap to humans.

Cleaning Up

Wash the affected area with alcohol immediately to lessen the rash. Combine the juice of two limes in one quart water mixed with equal parts white oak bark tea. This solution should be applied with a wet cloth or bandage and changed when it dries out. It should reduce healing time and severity of the attack.

Soap is a wonderful remedy for taking care of poison ivy or oak— before the rash appears. After contact with the plants, be sure to scrub the exposed area with soap to wash off the resin. Getting the resin off your skin is important—it will keep you from breaking out in a rash. Thoroughly washing the area within one to two hours of exposure should alleviate the problem before it starts. Any kind of soap should work fine, but some people swear by a brand called Fels-Naptha. I recommend scrubbing with this soap before going into an area where the plants are known to be, then scrubbing again after you return.

Some people find that household bleach helps to remove poison ivy or oak resin. First, wash the area well with a soap like Fels-Naptha. Then, soak a cotton ball in a half water, half bleach mixture and dab it on the area. Do this three times the first day that you notice blisters and you should see a definite improvement. Bleach can be a skin irritant, so test a small area before you proceed.

Herb Help

The herb goldenseal has been reported to relieve symptoms in just a few hours and even cure the rash in a day. Make a paste or purchase the liquid form for the fastest results.

Here's a hot idea that MUST be used cold. During the summertime, when poison ivy poses the biggest problem, make a batch of mugwort tea and keep it in a jar or bottle in the refrigerator until needed. As soon as you real-ize you've come in contact with the poi-son ivy, grab the refrigerated tea and wash your skin with it. If applied soon enough after the contact, mugwort tea can rid your skin of the rash-causing oil—but only if the tea is cold. Hot tea will open your pores and make the rash worse.

Friendly Foods

If poison ivy or oak is driving you bananas—this is the perfect cure for you. Peel a banana and set aside the fruit. You'll only need the peel for this remedy. Rub the inside of the skin on your rash every hour for one whole day. Use a new banana peel for each application. If you're lucky, someone you know will have a banana bread recipe as good as my Grandma's.

Placing tofu directly on a poison ivy rash can stop the itching and feel very cooling and soothing. Keep tofu in place with gauze pads.

Oatmeal is a great remedy for all kinds of itchy skin ailments, but it's especially good on poison ivy and poison oak. Fill some fine netting (or a sock or old pantyhose) with oatmeal and put it in a bathtub that's filling with warm, not hot, water. Hot water will make the rash worse. Have a good long soak. For even more itch control, leave the oatmeal residue on a little while before rinsing off. For patches of poison ivy or oak, make a paste out of oatmeal and tepid water. Place it on the rash until the itching subsides.

Getting Muddy

If you're camping or away from home, try putting fresh mud on the poison ivy or oak. The mud will help to draw out the infection.

Fire With Fire

When I was young, it seemed I was always getting into trouble—and I would always pay for it. I used to love to play in the woods with my friends, but more often than not we'd run into some poison ivy or poison oak and one of us would soon be covered in an itchy red rash. Grandma had shown me what the offending plants looked like, but when you're a kid and just want to have fun, defensive botany just doesn't seem important.

Grandma's remedy for the rash caused by these harmful plants was to use another plant: jewelweed. Jewelweed is also known as impatiens or touch-me-nots. The plant often grows near poison ivy and poison oak. Grandma would boil up a few of the plants in a gallon of water and strain the plant matter out. She always had a jar of it handy in the summer—and she always made enough for me and my friends.

GETTING PAST THE ROUGH PATCHES: PSORIASIS

This is a skin disorder characterized by patches of silvery looking scales or reddish areas on knees, elbows or the waist. It may be triggered by stressful events or extreme nervousness and may be hereditary.

Cod liver oil in capsule form taken one to two times a day has had excellent results in alleviating the disease and relieving the symptoms. Giving up caffeine also has a positive effect.

From The Herb Garden

Birch bark has been used on eczema, psoriasis, and numerous other skin problems throughout the years. Make a tea by boiling about three tablespoons of the powdered bark in one quart water. Simmer for ten minutes with the heat on low and let stand one hour. Strain the mixture well and place on a cloth. Leave on the affected area for at least one to two hours.

Apply a poultice of yellow dock, chaparral, and goldenseal to soothe the affected area and improve healing time.

TURNING RED: RASH

Baby's Delicate Skin

Babies get rashes all the time and are easily remedied. Since diaper rash is caused by too much wetness, a common-sense solution is letting the baby's skin air dry before diapering. Both fresh air and sunlight are good for skin. A little airing out can help heal or prevent diaper rash.

If you don't have time for a good air drying, use your blow dryer. Make sure you keep the heat low and don't get the dryer too close to your child. After all, baby's skin is sensitive, and you don't want to exchange a rash for a burn.

A good diaper can help prevent diaper rash. Among disposables, use the super-absorbent varieties that keep moisture away from the skin. If you prefer cloth diapers, try double-diapering and leaving off the rubber pants.

Healing The Hurt

One of Grandma's sure-fire remedies for baby rash was to place a thin coating of egg white on the affected area. The egg white coats and protects the area and promotes healing.

Grandma kept cornstarch in her kitchen cupboard, and she would rub a little on baby's bottom to dry out skin and help soothe diaper rash. Of course, you can always use baby powder, but not talcum.

A variety of over-the-counter ointments can help protect your child's delicate skin. Many people swear by Desitin Ointment, while others prefer petroleum jelly or A and D Ointment. A diaper rash can become infected by yeast. If this is the case with your child, try an over-the-counter anti-fungal treatment, such as Gyne-Lotrimin, normally used for vaginal infections.

Don't Do Anything Rash

For a sweet remedy, try rubbing honey gently on the rash. Honey has a smooth, creamy texture, and it is well known for it's anti-bacterial properties.

Although this remedy won't cure the problem, you may find putting apple cider on the rash to be very soothing. It can also be used to alleviate the sting of a sunburn.

Try putting cornstarch on your rash. It will keep the rash free of moisture and can soothe the itching. One warning: you should not use corn starch if you are prone to yeast infections.

Ease prickly heat and other such rashes by rubbing the sensitive area with the inside of a watermelon rind.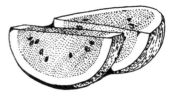

Soaking It In

Oatmeal is a terrific remedy for skin rashes. Put oats in a fine netting (try a sock or an old pair of pantyhose) and place in a warm bath. Soak in the tub for at least half an hour. Make sure the water is warm, not hot. Hot water can make rashes feel worse. An alternative to oatmeal is finely ground oats called colloidal oatmeal. You can find different brands of colloidal oatmeal at your pharmacy or in the bath section of your sundry store. Sprinkle the colloidal oatmeal in a tub filling with warm water. Soak for at least twenty minutes and carefully pat dry. You can take a colloidal oatmeal bath twice a day and it should relieve the discomfort of many common skin rashes.

Another bath additive you can try is dry mustard. Put a few table-spoons in a warm bath to soothe the itching and promote healing. My Grandma used to suggest our neighbor use this remedy when her husband would get prickly heat. Like the oatmeal bath, this bath will soothe the itching and keep you from scratching which is an important part of the healing process.

Don't Overreact

If you are prone to rashes on your hands, be wary of harsh deter-gents and dish washing liquids that can cause allergic reactions. Try switching to a non-allergenic brand for a few weeks. If your rash goes away, your old detergent was probably the culprit. To make sure, try the old detergent again. If the rash comes back, you have definitely found the cause of your discomfort. Some people with especially sensitive skin also get rashes from rubber gloves. If you suspect that this is the case, protect your hands by using vinyl gloves under your rubber gloves.

RING AROUND THE ROSY: RINGWORM

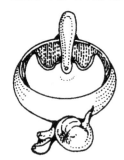

Ringworm responds to raw garlic placed over the ringworm under a Band-Aid.

OVEREXPOSED: SKIN CANCER

Skin cancers have been treated with tea prepared from chaparral. Place the tea in a poultice and apply for thirty minutes three times a day.

TOO MUCH OF A GOOD THING: SUNBURN

Excessive exposure of the bare skin to ultraviolet light for a prolonged period leads to burning.

Taking The Sting Out

Take the heat out of a sunburn quickly by applying apple cider vinegar to the burn. Put the vinegar in water to dilute it (try one part vinegar to two or three parts cool water) and apply it to the areas that are burned. That hot feeling you get from too much sun should disappear and the stinging sensation will subside. You may even find that applying the vinegar solution will keep you from peeling.

Cold clay poultices are very effective. Green tea that has been cooled and placed on the affected area with a washcloth will also have a soothing effect. The poultice should be left on for about thirty minutes every few hours.

Another soothing sunburn remedy is a cold milk compress. Put equal parts of milk and ice in a quart container and add about two tablespoons of salt. Soak a washcloth in the milky mixture and place it on the raw area. Leave the washcloth on for up to fifteen minutes and repeat three or four times during the day.

For a sunburned face, try spreading on yogurt or sour cream. Leave on for twenty minutes and let the yogurt or sour cream take the heat out of your burn. Rinse with lukewarm water.

Buttering Us Up

When one of us kids would come home "glowing like a firefly" from a nasty sunburn, Grandma would grab one of her handy kitchen helpers: butter. She would use the freshly churned variety. You may find that a can of evaporated milk will also do the trick. Milk has been known to ease a sunburn, but be sure to use whole milk. It's the fat content in the liquid that makes the raw skin feel better.

Don't Forget To Moisturize

Aloe vera gel does wonders for relieving the pain of sunburns and helps moisturize the skin. Many of today's commercial brands of sun care products claim aloe vera as one of the ingredients. If you have an aloe vera plant at home, cut off a leaf, break it open and spread the gel right on your burn. It's soothing and lubricating and helps in healing so you'll feel better in no time. If you don't have a plant handy, you can purchase aloe vera gel at your local health food store.

Another soothing solution for sunburns is vitamin E capsules. But in the case of a burn, you don't swallow it, you cut it open and spread the oil on the tender area. The oil will ease the pain of a sunburn and will also lubricate your skin to guard against peeling and blistering.

Grandma's Secret Anti-Wrinkle Lotion

My grandmother's skin always looked great. She hardly wrinkled despite her advancing years. Whenever anyone asked about her complexion, she would say, "Clean living is my secret." One day I saw her preparing a lotion from avocados, and she swore me to secrecy. It was the oil that was her secret. It makes one of the best suntan lotions. Avocado oil will also keep the skin in excellent condition and slow the skin's aging process.

Rub-A-Dub-Dub

Try taking a baking soda bath to relieve the pain of a sunburn. Sprinkle about a cup of baking soda into lukewarm water (careful, not too hot!) and soak for fifteen to twenty minutes. You might want to follow this up with one of the topical remedies.

Another bath additive good for sunburn pain is colloidal oatmeal. Look for colloidal oatmeal at you pharmacy or sundry store.

How about a milk bath to take the heat and sting away? Empty a package of powdered nonfat dry milk or a quart of low-fat milk into a tub of warm water. A half an hour soak should soothe away the sunburn pain.

The Eyes Have It

The delicate skin around the eye is very susceptible to sunburns. Tea bags are a good remedy for sunburned eyelids. Cool wet tea bags placed on the eyes will feel great and help in healing. Tea is also soothing for other sunburned skin. Try brewing a pot of strong tea, let it cool, and apply it on sunburned legs, arms, backs, etc.

Here's another eye-easing remedy. Prepare a poultice made from grated apples and place on your eyelids. Then lie back and relax—it will be helpful if you can keep the poultice on for about an hour.

Another good poultice for sunburned eyes is made by lightly beating one egg white. Wrap the poultice over your closed eyes and get a good night's sleep. Remove the poultice when you wake up and you should feel a noticeable improvement.

FROG PRINTS: WARTS

These are clusters of cauliflower-like growths that may appear anywhere on the body and are usually caused by a virus. They are contagious and should be isolated with a bandage and never irritated or picked.

Simple Medicine

Take two aspirin. . . another remedy for warts is aspirin. But you don't swallow it. Instead, dip your hand in warm water and place a damp aspirin tablet on the wart. Cover it with a Band-Aid or a gauze pad with tape to keep it in place. Put the aspirin on before going to bed. That one application should do the trick. Your wart should be history in just a few days. This remedy is not recommended for those who are allergic to aspirin.

Putting iodine on a wart several times a day can help to dissolve it away. Although this remedy may take a while, keep applying the iodine several times a day and the wart should fall off within a few weeks.

Here is a cure for plantar warts—the warts that appear on the soles of the feet. These warts can spread, so don't pick at them. Rub castor oil on the plantar wart each night before you go to bed. Keep this up until the wart's all gone.

Salt is also used as a cure for warts. Moisten some table salt and place it on the wart covering it with a Band-Aid. Keep this treatment up until the wart disappears.

Kitchen Cures

One of Grandma's remedies for warts was to strap on some black-strap molasses. Apply a poultice of the molasses and keep on as long as you can. She would also feed us a tablespoon of the blackstrap molasses each day. After about two weeks of the molasses treatment, the wart should drop right off.

Go figure—placing a crushed, fresh fig on the wart for a half hour each day will cause it to disappear. Be sure the fig is very mushy.

Try putting a used tea bag on the wart for fifteen minutes every day. Your wart should be toast in a week and a half.

Here's an egg cure—sort of. Soak your hand in the water from hard boiled eggs. Do this for ten minutes a day until the wart disappears. For some reason, this remedy works specifically for warts that appear on the hands.

Place crushed fresh garlic directly on the wart and cover with a dressing for a 24-hour period. The wart should develop a blister and eventually fall off. Castor oil has also been used with varied success.

Meadow-cine

Picking dandelions can have positive healing effects on warts. Break the dandelion off at the stem—a white, milky substance will appear. Put this on the wart several times a day until the wart goes away. Be careful, though. Dandelions may cause a rash for people with sensitive skin.

TURN BACK THE CLOCK: WRINKLES

The herb cleavers has been used as a facial cleanser and skin tightener with excellent results. It far outshadows most of the over-the-counter preparations that cost a small fortune. To prepare a mixture, bring one quart of pure filtered water to a boil. After removing the water from the heat, add three to four tablespoons of cleavers herb, then cover the mixture and allow it to steep for forty-five minutes. Apply the mixture by lightly saturating a small towel and placing it over your face for ten minutes three to four times a day for four days. The effects will remain for three to four weeks and will become evident in about two weeks.

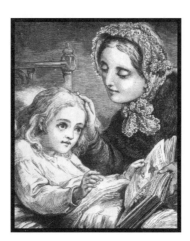

Chapter 2

BED-RIDDEN BLUES

STUCK WITH THE SNIFFLES: COLDS

Colds are caused by a virus, and the symptoms include various kinds of upper respiratory discomfort. Mucous should be allowed to flow freely, since the body rids itself of infection this way. The cold virus may take many forms making it difficult to fight.

A Few Tips On Prevention

"An ounce of prevention is worth a pound of cure." That was my grandmother's sage advice. Grandma recommended eating certain foods to help ward off colds and flus, and in fact, modern science has confirmed that there are benefits to eating more broccoli, parsley, and apples. The old adage that an apple a day keeps the doctor away may well be true! Grandma also recommended drinking raw sauerkraut juice every day to keep cold germs away. It has the added benefit of keeping you regular.

If someone at work has been coughing on you or one of your children has come down with a cold or the flu, take a cinnamon oil preventative immediately. Add five drops of cinnamon oil to a tablespoon of water and drink it down. Repeat three times a day. You can also take a teaspoon of eucalyptus oil to ward off a cold. Hold it in your mouth ten minutes before swallowing.

The shiitake mushroom has an important place in traditional Asian medicine. If you feel a cold coming on, add these tasty mushrooms to your favorite dish. Or you can take shiitake mushroom capsules if you prefer.

Tea And Sympathy

Grandma always said that when you've got the sniffles, something warm to drink and few soothing words went a long way to help the patient recover. Here are a few soothing suggestions:

Several herbal teas have a significant effect on cold symptoms. Goldenseal tea stands out as one of the best and is known to contain antibiotic properties.

Make a tea with cayenne pepper, just a pinch if you're not used to hot food. It can help prevent a cold or speed relief. The capsaicin in the pepper helps to loosen mucous.

Try this congestion curing tea. Make a mullein tea with two teaspoons dried leaves in one cup boiling water, steeping for ten minutes. The herb mullein can be found in health food stores. It helps soothe sore throats and breaks up mucous, easing congestion.

A tea made with slices of fresh ginger root or powdered ginger will help break up mucous and reduce fever. It may also boost the immune system.

Try this very-citrus cure that allows you to use your favorite liquor. In a saucepan, combine the juice of one orange, one lemon, and one grapefruit, along with a tablespoon of honey. Be sure to stir it while you bring it to a boil. Add an ounce or so of brandy or whatever you have on hand and enjoy.

Don't Knock Chicken Soup

Chicken soup works wonders. Heating the soup releases a chemical that relieves some of the symptoms, especially nasal drainage. Other foods that may also help are garlic, onions and hot peppers.

Drink a broth made from potato peels one to two times a day. The peels should be approximately a half inch thick and should include the skin. Clean the skin thoroughly with a good organic cleaner and a vegetable brush. Boil for twenty to thirty minutes with two stalks of celery. Cool and drink.

Don't Forget To Flush

Drinking a lot of water can help flush toxins and germs out of the body. You can also re-hydrate with unsweetened fruit juices and various kinds of herbal teas, including the ones mentioned here.

Rub It In And Breathe Deeply

Rub oil of eucalyptus into your chest two to three times a day. Breathing in this oil clears up congestion and opens airways. You can also place seven to eight drops of eucalyptus oil in hot bath water or six to seven drops in a cup of boiling water. Place a towel over your head and inhale the vapors.

If you have a chest cold, try rubbing a salve made from one raw egg white and four teaspoons prepared mustard into the chest. Apply a hot compress to the chest on top of the mixture and keep reapplying as the compresses get cold, four or five times. After the last one, wash off the salve and turn in for the night, making sure you don't get a draft. You should be able to sleep better and feel a lot less congested in the morning.

To clear out chest congestion, heat a cup of white wine and inhale the vapors.

Grandma's Cold Concoctions

Place one tablespoon of slippery elm bark powder in a half cup boiling water, add a quarter cup pure honey and the juice of half a lemon. Place the mixture in a jar and shake. Take one to two teaspoons every three hours.

My grandmother used the sunflower seeds she harvested from her garden to make a great cure for her family's colds. Follow her recipe by boiling a half cup sunflower seeds in five quarts of water, reducing the liquid by a little more than half. Add a quarter cup honey and three quarters cup gin. My grandmother instructed the cold-sufferer to take two teaspoons at each meal. Honey acts as an expectorant, and this remedy works especially well on a cold that is accompanied by a cough and chest congestion.

Grandma's Hot Dog Helper

Grandma used to say that the best way to lick a cold was a good old-fashioned "mustard plaster." She claimed this could cure almost any symptom. It is still used in many rural areas of the United States and Canada. To make the plaster, mash the leaves and stems of a fresh mustard plant into a thick pulp. Before applying the plaster, cover the chest with a thin layer of Vaseline. Put on the plaster and cover with a cloth or towel, taping it down. It is essential to protect skin with the Vaseline against any adverse effects of the mustard, such as blisters. For the best results, the plaster should be left on overnight. When grandma used the plaster, she would always make sure to tuck us in real good. By placing pillows on either side of us, she made sure we didn't move around too much during the night, keeping us "snug as a bug in a rug."

Smelly Solutions

Garlic appears to contain a substance that fights infections of all kinds: bacteria, viruses and fung-uses. It can help ward off or cure a cold. Fresh garlic is most effective, but you can also take dried garlic in the form of capsules or tablets.

Onions, like garlic, have traditionally been used to fight colds. If you're not an onion fan, look for onion preparations at your health food store.

Keep On Moving

When you come down with a cold, it makes you feel sluggish and your natural inclination is to rest. Grandma couldn't have disagreed more. She recommended getting out for a short walk, nothing too strenuous, just enough to get the blood going, bundling up if it was cold outside. In fact, it appears that exercise may stimulate the body's natural defenses to fight off infections.

A "Hard" Cure for Your Cold

Grandpa kept a flash of whiskey in the pie safe in the hallway. "Just for medicinal purposes," he always assured us. In fact, several traditional reme- dies for the common cold involve alcohol. Brew a mug of very strong black tea, add one tablespoon honey, one tablespoon cognac, one quarter teaspoon cinna- mon, and one teaspoon butter. The tea should be as hot as you can stand. You should wake up the next morning with soggy sheets, having sweat out the cold during the night.

If you prefer rum to cognac, try this remedy that combines the juice of one lemon and three teaspoons of honey with four teaspoons of rum. Before you go to bed, add the mixture to a glass of hot water and drink it down. You should feel much better in the morning.

Hot And Cold Cures

Soak in a hot tub that has ginger powder added to it, just before turning in for the night. Stay in the bath about fifteen minutes to get the full benefit. Make sure you dry off well afterwards to keep from getting chilled and dress warmly for bed. The ginger should help you sweat and rid the system of toxins. If the ginger does its job, you may have to change into a fresh, dry pair of pajamas during the night. By morning, you should feel noticeably better.

In traditional Chinese medicine, acupressure points are stimulated to relieve cold symptoms and cure the infection. Put a cube of ice on the bottom of each big toe, leaving in place until they melt. Do this three times a day until the cold clears up.

SOOTHING THE TICKLE: COUGHS

Soothing Solutions

Grandma's remedy for the common cough associated with a cold was hot tea with lemon and honey. The honey coats the throat and relieves the cough for a few hours. Another of her remedies was elderberry juice. Elderberry juice can calm the cough reflex for a long period of time. Fresh elderberries should be placed in a juicer with a slice of fresh lemon. Consume four to six ounces every three hours with a half teaspoon of honey or blackstrap molasses added as a sweetener.

Something Everyone Can Inhale

Put eucalyptus oil in a vaporizer and inhale the fumes.

Place ginger in very warm bath water. After the bath, wrap yourself in a terrycloth towel and sweat it out to loosen the mucous.

Peppermint, in its many forms, can be great for coughs. Put a drop of peppermint oil on your tongue to calm a coughing fit. Add a few drops of the oil to a cup of boiling water and inhale the vapors to relieve congestion. Make a tea of fresh peppermint leaves and drink with a little honey. You might even try a piece of peppermint candy. Grandma always had some in her purse, just in case.

If your congestion and cough is keeping you awake at night, take a warm bath before retiring, adding a couple of drops of pine oil to the water. The relaxing vapors should open up your bronchial passages and help you breathe more easily while you sleep.

Break It Up

Some hot spicy foods seem to help reduce the severity of a cough and break up the mucous and congestion usually associated with it. Try cayenne capsules, hot Chinese mustard and red horseradish. Apply hot onion packs to the chest and back at least three times a day. The onions should be sliced, steamed, and placed between soft cloths. Place a heating pad over the onion pack to help retain heat.

Control The Urge

Herbal cough drops help control the cough reflex. There are a number of effective herbs, such as eucalyptus and horehound.

Make a tea of slippery elm to get fast relief from a cough. You can buy lozenges with slippery elm as the active ingredient at your local health food store.

Throaty Solutions

A bay leaf poultice works wonders on chest congestion and coughing. Add twenty bay leaves to a cup of boiling water, cover and let stand for fifteen minutes. Put the warm, moist leaves in a cloth, placing it on your chest and covering with a towel to retain heat. Keep the liquid to re-freshen the bay leaves after an hour. Make sure you heat the water before soaking the leaves in it.

Gargle with a mixture of warm water and three tablespoons of dark Karo syrup. It will relieve a hacking cough.

Breakfast Breakthroughs

The fat in dairy products can help coat the throat and soothe a dry cough. Warm a cup of milk (not skim) and add two teaspoons of sweet butter. Drink two to three cups a day until the cough is gone. Milk contributes to the production of mucous, so you shouldn't try this remedy if you're coughing up phlegm or feel congested.

Certain ingredients in oatmeal can ease coughing. Make a thick oatmeal by following the directions on the package, reducing the water by a quarter cup. Flavor with honey to taste. Don't add milk to it, for the above reasons. Eat one cup of warm oatmeal, four times a day, or whenever the cough flares up.

A Honey Of A Cough Remedy

Grandma had a few "sweet" cures for a cough, involving honey. In the first, she combined six medium-sized onions, coarsely chopped, along with a half cup honey in the top of a double boiler. She simmered the mixture slowly for two hours and stored it in a tightly sealed jar. She'd warm it up and give the cough-sufferer a tablespoon every two to three hours. She made her other "sweet" cough cure from one teaspoon horseradish and two teaspoons of honey. She used the same dosage as her other honey remedy, one teaspoon every few hours.

Here's a tasty cough remedy you'll enjoy even when you're well. In a mug, combine the juice of a large lemon, two tablespoons of honey, three cloves, a half a cinnamon stick, and enough hot water to top off the cup. The steam will ease your congestion, and the lemony warmth will soothe your throat. Take a mug every three hours to relieve an irritating cough.

Use root vegetables and something sweet to stop a persistent cough. Cut the middle out of a rutabaga or yellow onion and fill with brown sugar or honey. Leave overnight and drink the juice in the morning. You can also take a beet and cut a hole in it. Add brown sugar or honey and bake until it's soft. It's a tasty way to knock out a cough. A turnip will also work.

Barley Makes It Better

Sometimes I dream about my grandmother's beef barley soup. That's how good it was. Although I have the recipe, it never tastes quite the same when I make it. Grandma was simply magic in the kitchen. When someone in the family had been hacking for a few days, she'd make a big pot of her soup and whip up a cough remedy while she was at it. She'd add the juice of one lemon to a cup of cooked barley and liquefy it. She'd give the cougher a cup of her barley brew, advising them to drink it slowly, every four hours.

Liquor Is Quicker

Mulled wine was the beverage of choice in merry, old England, especially around the holidays. Add a cinnamon stick, three cloves, a tablespoon of honey, and a few pieces of lemon peel to three cups dry red wine. Make sure you stir while heating and try not to splash onto countertops since the red wine can stain. Take up to three cups a day. It should help relieve coughing, but even if it doesn't, you'll feel much happier.

Just one sip of whiskey should relax the cough reflex. Many commercial cough syrups contain alcohol.

Homemade Cough Syrups

Try these folksy recipes for cough syrup: Combine the juice of one lemon, a half cup olive oil, and one cup honey and cook for five minutes. Remove from heat and stir for several minutes. Take one teaspoon every two hours. Or mix a half cup water with a half cup apple cider vinegar, adding one teaspoon cayenne pepper and enough honey to sweeten for your individual taste. Take a tablespoon at

• *Bed-Ridden Blues* •

bedtime and anytime you have a severe coughing fit.

For a dry cough, boil three unpeeled potatoes. Retain the warm water and sweeten with honey. Take a tablespoon whenever you feel a coughing fit coming on.

Get some fresh ginger root and cut off a small piece. Wash and chew on it, swallowing the juice. This should help soothe your throat and ease your cough. Ginger root is a little pungent for some people's taste. If it's too strong for you, try one of the other remedies.

Boiled Bean Cough Cure

It doesn't seem that eating mashed up kidney beans should help relieve a cough, but Grandma relied on her Boiled Bean Cure for the worst of the worst, those deep, persistent coughs that nothing seems to help. Soak the kidney beans over night to soften. In the morning, drain off the water and tie up the beans in some plastic wrap or a tea towel. Beat the beans with whatever is handy, a sauce pan or bowl. Boil the bruised beans in two cups of water, along with three cloves of minced garlic, for about two hours, until they are soft. Make sure you watch the level of liquid and add more water if the beans get too dry. Whenever you have a coughing fit, eat a tablespoon of the beans.

Cure By The Cupful

A speedy cure for a bad cough is a warm cup of dill tea. Make the brew from one teaspoon of dill and a cup of boiled water. Let it stand for seven minutes before straining it. If you don't like the taste, sweeten it with a teaspoon or two of honey. Drink three cups throughout the day. If the cough isn't gone, repeat the next day, but you probably won't need to.

• Bed-Ridden Blues •

If you've had a cough so long it feels like you were born with it and you think you may have pulled a muscle in your back from all the endless hacking, it's time to take this powerful herbal remedy—fenugreek. On the first day, drink a cup of fenugreek tea every hour or so. Reduce the dosage the next day to four cups spread evenly throughout the day. You should be able to feel the chest congestion breaking up, and the cough should soon fade away. Since fenugreek is such strong medicine, only turn to this remedy when the others you've tried have failed and your cough is very persistent.

Licorice root has long been a staple in traditional healing. It is especially effective in treating upper respiratory ailments, including sore throats, colds, and coughing. Brew a tea from the licorice root or look for tea bags at your local health food store.

Grandma's Sunflower Cough Syrup

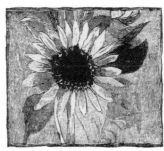

My grandmother often turned to her garden for her home remedies. Every year, she planted a row of beautiful sunflowers on one end of the garden, next to the peas, and at the end of the season, she would harvest the seeds and keep them on hand for snacks and cures. To treat a cough, she would whip up her Sunflower Cough Syrup. She'd cook a half cup of the seeds in five cups of water, boiling it down to about two cups of liquid. She'd strain out the seeds and add about a half cup of honey. She would get Grandpa's bottle out of the piesafe in the hall, whatever he happened to have on hand "for medicinal purposes," usually whiskey, and add some of that to her cough syrup, about three quarters cup as far as I could see. She would stir it all up and seal it tightly in a bottle. She would give the cough sufferer a teaspoon or two, four times a day. When you make this at home, you can use any hard liquor you happen to have on hand.

IT'S HOTTER THAN HECK IN HERE: FEVER

Normal body temperature ranges between 98 and 99 degrees Farenheight. If your fever is over 102 degrees Farenheight, you should consult a physician.

Fevers affect zinc absorption, so avoid supplements containing this mineral. Lobelia extract reduces fevers. Take a half teaspoon every three to four hours. If stomach discomfort occurs, reduce the dose to a quarter teaspoon.

Cool It

Fevers respond well to rubbing alcohol placed on the feet, palms and wrists. This increases evaporation through the skin and creates a cooling effect for the entire body.

Evaporation helps cool the blood. If you're running a fever, try taking a cool bath or shower, splash your face with cool water, or apply a cold compress to your forehead or wrists.

Out Of The Frying Pan

Heat can also cure a fever by inducing a therapeutic sweat. Take a hot bath or lie in bed under lots of warm quilts. Once you start perspiring, come out from under the blankets and let your sweat evaporate which will help cool the blood. Don't work out to cause sweating, and be sure to drink plenty of liquids.

Teas, in many varieties, have long been used to reduce fevers. The warmth will help induce a sweat. Brew a cup of black tea, add some sugar or honey, let cool for a minute, and slip in an ice cube. Sip slowly while resting in bed. Take a second cup if needed.

A Grape Idea

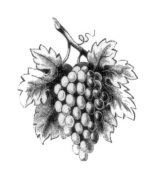

Try eating grapes throughout the day to relieve a fever. You can also drink pure, unsweetened grape juice, preferably diluted, always at room temperature, never chilled.

Put It On

For a homespun fever remedy, soak a folded piece of brown paper bag in white vinegar and place on the forehead.

Fry up some onions and put them in a bag or pillow case. Place it on the chest layered between towels and put a heating pad on top. This should cause sweating which will help break the fever. You can also put onion slices in your socks before bedtime, and the fever should be gone in the morning.

Drink It Up

Lemon balm has proven an effective fever remedy for Grandma and many other home healers. Steep leaves in boiling water to make a tea, and add lemon and honey. Two or three cups should help break a fever.

Grandma's "Fishy" Fever-Beater

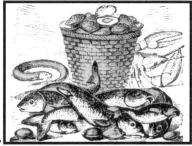

Grandma swore by cod liver oil. The rest of us swore that it tasted really awful, so she tried to mix it with other things to help it go down more easily. Mix up a batch of Grandma's Fever Beater with two or three tablespoons of lemon juice, a half teaspoon cod liver oil, and honey to taste. Remember cod liver oil is strong tasting stuff, so go easy on it.

DOWN FOR THE COUNT: FLU

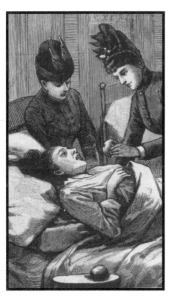

This highly contagious viral infection usually affects the respiratory tract. It is spread through the air and tends to change strains, making it difficult to cure.

Tea For Flu

Yarrow tea has positive effects in reducing the severity of symptoms. Catnip tea enemas reduce fevers.

Try a tea made from echinacea or ginger, sipped slowly every three to four hours.

A Spoonful Of Relief

The fruit of the gooseberry plant is called "alma" or "amalaki." One alma contains more Vitamin C than seven oranges. Take one to two teaspoons of alma a day if you think you have the flu. It should lessen the effects and boost the body's immune response.

Take one tablespoon blue or black elderberries in syrup form three times a day. This syrup is available in most health food stores. In recent years, studies have been done in Israel on this remedy.

In One Nostril And Out The Other

In our family the flu would spread like wild fire. Grandma used to make us use a nasal wash to keep the sinuses free of the virus. To make the wash: Use a half teaspoon of fennel seed in one cup of water and allow to simmer for ten minutes. Add an eighth teaspoon of sea salt and cool the mixture to room temperature. Drain out all the fennel seeds and place the mixture in a "neti pot." Lean your head over the sink and tilt it to one side. Pour a half of the mixture into one nostril; it will come out the other side. Then pour the balance into the other nostril.

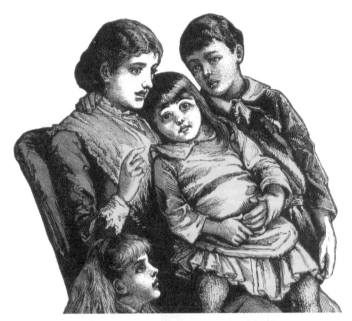

WHEN IT HURTS TO SWALLOW: SORE THROAT

This ailment may be caused by an environmental irritant or infection. It is a severe irritation of the mucous membrane at the back of the throat.

Here's a note about prevention: During the cold and flu season, it's important to be aware that germs can spread. Make sure to wipe telephones, door handles and other shared surfaces—even the television remote—with a disinfectant spray. You can also use Lysol Disinfectant Spray on pillowcases and bed linens to keep sick family members from re-infecting themselves.

Grandma's Works-Every-Time Tea

Grandmother had a great remedy for sore throats. This tea made from fresh hyssop works wonders. To prepare the tea, place two to three teaspoons of the dried herb in a cup of boiling water and allow to steep for ten to twelve minutes. Two or three cups a day should help relieve the problem.

Grandma's Gargles

Whenever I had a sore throat, my grandmother had me gargle with salt water. She would put about a teaspoon or two of salt water into lukewarm water and stir it up. I say about a teaspoon or two because when it came to measurements for cooking and baking, my grandmother's measuring technique was by sight, not science. She would hand me a glass of the salty water several times during the day and night, until I started feeling better.

Try gargling with a solution of a half teaspoon of sea salt with a small amount of chlorophyll added every hour. For that annoying feeling of post nasal drip, Grandma would use a vinegar and water gargle. She claimed that it cut the excess mucous in the back of the throat. Take about a tablespoon of apple cider vinegar in a glass of lukewarm distilled water and gargle. Sometimes, the vinegar would sting my throat. Then Grandma would use the honey and lemon remedy instead.

Another good gargle for a sore throat is hydrogen peroxide. Gargling with the solution three times a day should bring relief. I recommend mixing water with a three percent hydrogen peroxide solution and gargling about three times a day.

One way to get rid of laryngitis is an apple cider vinegar one-two punch. Mix two teaspoons of apple cider vinegar in one glass of lukewarm water. Gargle the first mouthful and spit it out, then swallow the next. Repeat this pattern until you've finished the glass. You can repeat this every hour. Many people have found they can be heard again after about seven doses. This remedy can also be good for sore throats, but you will probably only need to repeat this "vinegar gargle swallow" for two or three hours and you'll notice a difference.

Nothing To Sneeze At

This is a remedy that may sound strange, but give it a try. Put some cayenne pepper in ginger ale. This won't get high marks for flavor, but both the cayenne and the ginger have properties that will lubricate and heal the throat.

Sweet And Sour Solutions

Another of Grandmother's sore throat remedies was honey and lemon. Take a tablespoon of honey and squeeze some lemon on it (reconstituted lemon juice will do). Then, lean back and drizzle it down the back of your throat. I don't think this went a long way toward the healing of the sore throat, but it got rid of the persistent scratchy feeling long enough for me to fall asleep. And as far as remedies go, honey and lemon is very easy to take—especially for children.

A tea made from raw honey and lemon juice will help soothe the affected area. Honey is the only food that will not grow bacteria. Plus coating the throat with honey will reduce the level of bacterial growth and speed healing.

Grandma's Garden Variety Cure

Among the plants in Grandmother's herb garden was one she relied on for the cough and sore throat season: hyssop. She told us how her grandmother would brew her a cup of the soothing tea when she was a little girl. Hyssop makes an excellent tea for easing the coughing that can irritate a sore throat. Two teaspoons of dried herb should do the trick. Steep in boiling water for several minutes. If you have fresh hyssop on hand, steep the herb longer, but use the tea more sparingly. Tea in general is good for the throat, the heat is soothing, and drinking a lot of liquids is always recommended to keep the throat lubricated. Hot liquids can help to unstuff your nose.

Cures For Suckers

One way to numb a sore throat is to suck on a clove. It will be hot, but hold it in your mouth and let it warm your throat. It will also help to lubricate your throat to ease dryness. Try doing this before bedtime to ease the discomfort and let you fall asleep. Be careful not to swallow the clove; clove can upset your stomach.

If sucking on a clove doesn't appeal to you, try zinc lozenges. Many people swear by this remedy and claim that the zinc lozenges won't just get rid of your sore throat, it can also get rid of your cold. Try this remedy for yourself and decide. You'll find zinc lozenges in your local health food store.

Tea You Don't Swallow

When you have a sore throat it is important to get lots of rest and drink lots of liquids (but make sure you don't drink any dairy). And while drinking herbal tea can help you feel much better, here's another way that chamomile tea can give you relief. Brew some chamomile tea and let it cool just enough for you to be able to handle the heat. Soak a white towel in it, wring it out and place it on your throat. Once the towel loses its heat, dip it in the tea again, wring it out and reapply.

• *Bed-Ridden Blues* •

Here's a tea you gargle with, but don't swallow. Steep three tea bags in a cup of boiling water—use the non-herbal kind—until the tea is very, very dark. Let cool slightly and gargle with the still hot beverage. Remember, don't swallow. Repeat this every hour until you begin to feel better.

Put The Hoarse Out To Pasture

Try this remedy for hoarseness. Slowly boil a half cup of anise seed in one cup of water for fifty minutes. Strain the anise seed, and while still hot add a quarter cup of raw honey and one tablespoon of cognac. Take one tablespoon every half an hour.

Grandma's Vampire Vapors

Here's a remedy that is wonderful for the throat but not so appealing to the nose: garlic. Grandma knew that garlic had a lot of wonderful properties, and whenever she felt "a tickle on the creep" she would reach for the garlic, saying that it cleared her sinuses and helped her throat. Grandma would either put a garlic clove in her mouth or rub garlic oil on her neck. Neither of these remedies is recommended if you're expecting company, but Grandma swore that her smelly solution did the trick.

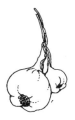

Chapter 3

SEE NO EVIL, HEAR NO EVIL, SMELL NO EVIL

CLEAR THE CANAL: EAR INFECTION

Ear infections cause pressure to increase in the outer or middle ear. The canal becomes inflamed and swelling occurs. It may cause a temporary loss of hearing in the affected ear. These infections are very painful for both adults and children. A physician should be consulted.

Earache "Don'ts"

"Don't go out of this house without a hat!" Grandma would say to us in the winter. It was good advice. The ears can be extremely sensitive to cold. Sometimes only a little chill or a strong wind can make them ache. Take care of your ears by wearing a hat, scarf or ear muffs.

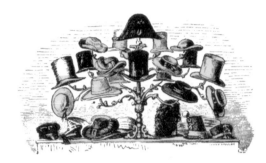

If you have an earache, avoid forceful nose blowing that can push mucous further back into the sinuses and into the passage between the throat and ears.

Sit Up Straight

Just sitting up can help reduce the pain and congestion of an ear ache. Elevating the head helps clear the passages that run between the throat and middle ears, equalizing pressure.

Warming Trends

Heat is one of the best soothers for an earache. Put a washcloth in a bowl of water and microwave for forty-five seconds. Hold it against your sore ear. Then direct the airflow from your blow dryer into your sore ear, keeping if far enough away so that your skin and hair don't get burned.

Fill a handkerchief or clean sock with a quarter cup table salt. Wrap a rubber band around it to make a ball and warm in the oven on low-heat. Lie down with the compress against your ear. The heat should bring relief from the pain. Some people claim this remedy works better if you add a quarter cup raw bran to the salt.

If your child has an ear ache, try the hug remedy. Put one hand over one ear and press the other into your chest. Your body's warmth will make the ache better.

Splish, Splash, Don't Do Anything Rash

Getting water in your ear while swimming or showering can be very annoying. If you have a problem with swimmer's ear, put a few drops of jojoba or mineral oil in your ears before diving in.

Stick It In Your Ear

There are a number of substances that can be placed in the ear to relieve pain. Buy garlic oil capsules at your local health store. Poke a hole in one of the capsules and let the oil drip into your ear. Seal the ear with a cotton ball. The pain should begin to diminish within half an hour. You can also try mixing together four drops of onion juice and one teaspoon warm olive oil. Place in the ears the same way as above, making sure to plug the ears with cotton. Apply three drops to each ear, in the morning and evening.

Alleviate pain by placing a few drops of warm olive oil in the ear along with a drop of tincture of lobelia. Children who live around smokers tend to have more frequent ear infections. This method should not be used before seeing a physician, since it will cause problems if the eardrum has been perforated.

If the idea of putting something into your ear canal makes you uncomfortable, try this remedy instead. Put some castor oil on a cotton ball and add a little black pepper. Place on the outside of the ear to relieve pain.

Grandma's Russian Remedy

My grandmother called this cure for an earache her Russian Remedy, since it involves vodka, something she only allowed into the house for medicinal purposes. I had a terrible time with earaches when I was little, as many children do. She'd get out her medicine dropper and the vodka, and gently put a couple of drops, no more than four, into my ear. I don't think it was ever longer than five minutes before my ear felt much better.

SILENCE IS GOLDEN: RINGING EARS

It may affect one or both ears and can be caused by poor carbohydrate metabolization. Fluid retention in the semicircular canals, or wax build-up, may also cause ringing in the ears.

Quit It

Sometimes, if you have a terrible headache, you may take more than the recommended dose of aspirin or other analgesics. These over-the-counter drugs contain substances that can cause your ears to ring. Stop taking the drug, and the ringing should stop when it wears off.

For persistent ringing in the ears that is not caused by medication, take fenugreek tea, three times a day, in the morning, afternoon, and before going to bed. To make the tea, add a teaspoon of fenugreek seeds to a cup of boiling water, steeping for twenty minutes. It will take a couple of weeks to be effective.

Get Rid Of Waxy Buildup

Earwax is often the culprit when you have ringing in the ears. To get rid of the buildup, put a teaspoon of warm (not hot!) sesame oil into each ear, and seal with cotton balls. Let it work for a couple of minutes to loosen the wax, then take out the cotton and wash out your ears. An easy way to wash out the ears is to take a shower and let the water stream into the ears. Both the oil and wax will flow out. Hopefully, the ringing will be a thing of the past. You can also use castor oil in much the same way to cure chronic ringing in the ears.

To remove ear wax, place a few drops of warm olive oil in the ear and seal with a piece of cotton while keeping your head tilted to the side. Remove the cotton and add a few drops of hydrogen peroxide. The oil will soften the wax and the bubbling action of the hydrogen peroxide will loosen the wax and carry it out.

To clear out earwax that can contribute to ringing ears, fill a syringe with warm water. Gently squirt the water into the ear, and the wax will come out in a few minutes. Of course, you should always be careful when dealing with the ears.

Dip a cotton ball in warm oil that has been sprinkled with black pepper. Place carefully in the ear and leave for five minutes to reduce ear wax that can cause ringing in the ears.

Hot Blooded

Problems with blood supply and circulation can contribute to ringing in the ears. To redistribute blood flow and get rid of the ringing, put a heating pad on your hands and feet.

Stick It In Your Ear

My grandmother believed in onion juice as the cure for ringing ears. Place two drops in your ears, repeating three times a week.

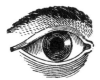 # EYE PROBLEMS

These may include the eyes becoming bloodshot, a burning sensation, general irritation, sensitivity to light, or blurred vision. Nicotine from smoking, high sugar intake and excess coffee drinking may affect a person's vision.

The herb eyebright has been used for centuries for many eye problems with great success. It may be taken as a tea or capsule form. If eyebright is not available, goldenseal may be substituted.

SEEING RED: BLOODSHOT EYES

The best way to treat anything is to get to the root of the problem. Bloodshot eyes can be caused by lack of sleep or too much hard drinking. If you have this problem and neither of these causes fits the bill, you may have a vitamin deficiency. Try taking a supplement of B-2, according to your doctor's instructions, or take brewer's yeast, an excellent source of B vitamins.

A Spicy Solution

Grandma recommended this old, country cure using ginger to treat bloodshot eyes. She'd make a wet paste out of two tablespoons ginger and a little water. She'd have the person put the paste on the soles of their feet, pull on a thick pair of socks to save the sheets, and have them turn in for bed. When they woke up in the morning, you could see the whites of their eyes.

HOW MANY FINGERS?: BLURRED VISION

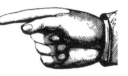

If you have a problem with blurred vision, treat it with alfalfa. At your local health food store, look for alfalfa tablets. In a cup of boiled water, thoroughly dissolve one tablet. Cool and strain the mixture, and store it in a tightly sealed bottle. Use the solution for eyedrops, one drop in each eye daily, preferably in the morning. It should help clear up your eyesight.

IN THE PINK: CONJUNCTIVITIS

To treat conjunctivitis, or pink eye, grate an apple or raw red potato and make up a poultice. Close your eyes and apply the poultice for at least thirty minutes. The pink eye should clear up within two or three days.

Chamomile tea makes a fine eyewash to treat conjunctivitis. Bathe your eyes twice a day until the conditions heals. You can also use fennel tea to wash your eyes. Steep a teaspoon of fennel seeds in a cup of boiling water for five minutes. Strain out the seeds and let it cool before using it. If your eyes are irritated, put a couple of drops of milk or castor oil into each eye.

I CAN SEE CLEARLY NOW: EYESIGHT

It sounds like a cliche, but drinking carrot juice can help improve your eyesight. Take a small glass, twice a day. Soon, you'll be seeing better than ever.

Chew On This

My grandmother's favorite snack was fresh sunflower seeds harvested from her garden. She had remarkable eyesight for a woman her age. As it happens, sunflower seeds contain many nutrients that are good for the eyes. Make them a staple of your diet, eating a half cup every day.

Traditional Asian healers recommend ginger to strengthen eyesight. Chew a piece after every meal.

GET SOME SHUT EYE: EYESTRAIN

If you spend a lot of your day reading or staring into a computer screen, you probably suffer from eyestrain. Traditional Chinese medicine prescribes acupressure to relieve tired eyes. Pinch the center of your index and middle fingers, thirty seconds on each finger. Your eyes should feel refreshed in a matter of minutes. If not, repeat the procedure.

REST FOR THE WEARY: IRRITATED AND TIRED EYES

Keep Them Covered

To beat eye irritation, peel an over-ripe apple and place the flesh on your closed eyes. Use gauze or cloth to keep it in place and leave on for thirty minutes.

There are several poultices than can be applied to the eyes to reduce irritation and inflammation. Try

81

grated Irish potato, papaya pulp, or cooked, mashed beets. Apply twice a day and leave on for at least fifteen minutes.

There are several herbs that can be used on compresses to soothe tired and irritated eyes. Make fennel tea by steeping a tablespoon of fennel seeds in two cups of boiling water. Allow it to steep for fifteen minutes and then apply with cotton or cloth. You can also use the herb horsetail. Measure out a teaspoon and steep in boiling water for ten minutes. Leave the warm compress on for ten minutes at a time and keep re-wetting the cotton until your eyes are soothed.

Close your weary eyes and apply a warm compress of rosemary tea to soothe and refresh. You can use fresh rosemary, the dried herb, or tea bags. Let it steep for ten minutes in boiling water. Soak some cotton or a cloth in the tea, put it on your eyelids, and relax for ten minutes or more.

European Eye Cup Cure

The herb chervil has been used for severe eye inflammation in Europe. Prepare the herb by placing a quarter cup diced leaves in one cup boiling water, boil five minutes and remove from the heat. Allow to cool to body temperature and apply the mixture in an eye cup.

Just Resting My Eyes

Sometimes, Grandma's common sense points out things that should be obvious, but somehow manage to elude us anyway. Grandma always said that if you were tired you should rest. She believed the same was true if your eyes were tired. When I'd spent too much time going over homework and my eyes were bothering me, she'd send me into the front room to lie down, to rest or nap for twenty minutes or so. I'd get up feeling fresh, ready to wrestle with my long division once more.

DON'T FLIP YOUR LID: STYS

Tea Treatments

To cure a sty, brew a tea with a handful of parsley leaves in a cup of boiling water, allowing to steep for ten minutes. Soak a washcloth in the tea, lie down, close your eyes, and place it over your eyes for fifteen minutes. Also try this remedy on puffy eyes.

If you have a sty on your eye, save the tea bag from your afternoon cup of tea. Apply to your closed eye with gauze or cloth before going to bed and leave over night. The sty should be gone in the morning. You need to use black tea, not herbal, to get the right active ingredients.

Swab It Away

Simply swabbing a sty with a little castor oil on a piece of cotton can help clear it up in a matter of days.

Fools Gold?

One of the most popular folk remedies for a sty is to rub it with a gold wedding ring. This may fall more into the category of superstition than science, but what could it hurt to give it a try?

LOSE THE LUGGAGE: UNDER-EYE PUFFINESS

If you tend to wake up with under-eye puffiness, brew yourself a cup of black tea, enjoy, and wait for the tea bags to cool. Close your eyes and apply. Pretty soon, your eyes should look much less puffy. The gentle acid in the tea causes the tissues to contract.

In old movies, you'll sometimes see a starlet relaxing with cool slices of cucumber on her closed eyelids. It's a great way to refresh tired eyes and can also help reduce under-eye puffiness.

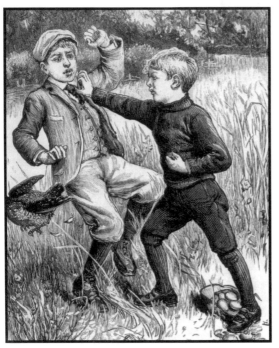

NOSEBLEEDS

Nosebleeds may be caused by an injury or excessive dryness that causes the delicate nasal blood vessels to rupture. Sudden changes in atmospheric pressure will also cause these small vessels to break.

Giving It Lip Service

Putting a wad of paper, cotton or gauze inside your mouth between your top lip and gum may help to slow and eventually stop the bleeding.

You may also try putting pressure on the outside of your upper lip. Place a strip of cardboard or paper between your upper lip and nose and press firmly. This is an effective remedy that works with known acupressure points. Press firmly, squeezing for about a minute or so, and your nosebleed should stop.

In A Pinch

Pinch the center of your nose (just below the bony part) with your thumb and forefinger. Keep pinching for several minutes, and your nosebleed should stop.

Hot And Sour Stoppers

Here's a hot tip: drink a glass of warm water with an eighth teaspoon of cayenne pepper added. It should stop the bleeding.

Vinegar can help get a nosebleed under control. Wash the temples, nose and neck with a cloth that's been soaking in vinegar. In addition, drink a half glass of water with two teaspoons of vinegar mixed in.

Grandma's Silver Dollar Nosebleed Stopper

Grandma had a special treatment when one of us kids got a nosebleed. To stop the bleeding, she'd reach for her magic silver dollar which she kept in the freezer for such occasions. She'd press it on the back of our necks and just like magic, the bleeding would stop. Grandma's other chilly solution for nosebleeds was reserved for the adults— but both worked equally well. First she would make the person sit up with the head tilted down (you can tilt it back if you like, but the blood will run down your throat and may cause a stomach ache—either way, just make sure that your head is above your heart). Then she either wrapped ice in a dish towel and place it on the back of the neck. It always seemed to help. Ice packs work well, too.

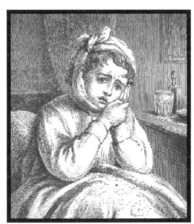

Chapter 4

WELL, SHUT MY MOUTH!

SLAYING THE DRAGON: BAD BREATH

Bad breath is usually caused by improper dental hygiene, digestive tract problems or smoking. It may be a sign of poor overall health.

Brush Away Bad Breath

Change your new tooth brush every two months to avoid bacteria buildup. Try brushing your teeth and tongue with myrrh at least twice a week.

• *Well. Shut My Mouth!* •

Baking soda is a fine old standby to use in place of toothpaste. It is abrasive enough to clean and whiten the teeth, as well as to keep bad breath away.

Brushing your tongue is a must if you have a problem with bad breath. Bacteria remain in the small deep pores in the tongue and must be brushed out. Baking soda works well for tongue brushing.

Grandma's Breathalizer

If there was one thing Grandma wouldn't stand for, it was bad breath. She always had a remedy handy for those of us who didn't pass her approval. You never refused when she told you to wash out your mouth. Here's the recipe for her homemade mouthwash: Place ten tablespoons of fresh powdered cinnamon in one and a quarter cups of inexpensive vodka. Add sufficient water to dilute the alcohol to a fifty percent solution. Place the mixture in a jar and allow it to stand for two weeks. Seal the jar well and shake it twice a day, once in the morning and once at night. After two weeks, strain the mixture into a clean jar and store in a cool place. Grandma always kept hers in the bathroom. When you use the mixture just add a half teaspoon to four ounces of water and swish it around several times in your mouth. Don't swallow—or you may fail a different Breathalizer test!

Chew On This

Chewing a small amount of parsley will correct most breath problems. Peppermint also contains cleansing properties.

For millennia, people have been chewing cloves to sweeten their breath. Give it a try yourself. Could all those people have been wrong for all that time?

You know how much cleaner your mouth feels after chewing a piece of Big Red? For a natural breath sweetener without added sugar, chew on a cinnamon stick. Also try chewing anise seeds. You'll especially enjoy this breath freshener if you like the taste of licorice.

Beat Bad Breath With Good Nutrition

Since poor overall health and bad nutrition can contribute to breath problems, try adding more fruits and vegetables to your diet, especially apples, green leafy vegetables, and psyllium (an ingredient in laxatives like Metamucil).

The next time you go out for Italian food and come back with garlic breath, suck on a lemon. It also works for onion breath. Some people believe this cure works better if you put salt on the lemon.

A Cup Of Fresh Breath

My grandmother was a big coffee drinker, and she made the best coffee you can imagine. To get rid of onion breath, she prescribed a cup of strong, black coffee. For friends and neighbors who didn't drink coffee, she recommended eating an apple to counteract oniony bad breath. Now that I think of it, she would eat an apple to freshen coffee breath. Maybe Grandma would have skipped the coffee treatment and just eaten an apple in the first place if she hadn't enjoyed a good, warm cup so much.

SOOTHING THE SENSITIVE SMILE: BLEEDING GUMS

Cut a small strip of lemon peel and wrap it around your finger so the white rind faces out. Rub the white area on the sore gum for five minutes, two to three times a day. The bleeding should stop, and the gums should heal within a week. You should also consume two fresh oranges a day.

PUTTING OUT THE FIRE: BURNING MOUTH

A number of spices will react unfavorably with the mouth's delicate tissues, causing a painful burning hot sensation and even damage. One of the more common spices that causes this reaction is cayenne, found in a variety of peppers. Grandma had two cures for this problem and both seem to work equally well. To quench the fire, try drinking either whole milk or beer. The chemical that causes the hot bite is capsaicin which dissolves easily in either fat or alcohol.

A MOUTH FULL OF TROUBLE: CANKER SORES

These sores are caused by bacterial contamination, a virus, or certain foods that irritate the mouth.

Pucker Up

When one of us kids got a canker sore, Grandma would have us eat as many pickles as we could. Alum, one of the pickling ingredients, will dry up the area which promotes healing and relieves pain. You can also put a little alum directly on a sore. You can find alum in the spice section of your local supermarket.

Swish, Swash But Don't Swallow

Treat canker sores with hydrogen peroxide diluted with water. Swish around in the mouth two to three times a day, making sure none is swallowed, to kill the bacteria. Be careful not to overuse, or it will kill friendly bacteria as well. Because bacteria thrive in warm, moist environments, a canker sore will take about ten days to heal if left untreated.

Washing your mouth out with very strong, warm salt water three or four times a day can help take away canker sore pain and speed healing. The salt may sting, but it should clear up the sore in a couple of days.

Aloe vera gel can take the pain out of canker sores, just as it does burns. Rinse your mouth out with aloe vera gel the way you would mouthwash, several times a day, until the condition clears up. You can find aloe vera gel at your local health food store. Aloe vera appears to have anti-bacterial properties.

Swishing some Mylanta around your mouth may speed healing of a canker sore. Don't swallow unless you also have an upset stomach.

What The Milk Man Knows

Drinking a glass of milk can help your canker sore feel better. Swish a little milk or buttermilk around your mouth three or four times a day to reduce pain.

Yogurt and acidophilus contain good bacteria that may fight off the bad bacteria that cause canker sores. To prevent sores in the first place, eat a little yogurt every day.

Dab It On To Dry It Up

Place a pinch of baking soda on your sore to dry it up. You can also make a paste by adding a little water to one teaspoon baking soda. Place on the canker sore and keep reapplying when it dissolves. Baking soda helps fight bacteria, and brushing your teeth with baking soda may help prevent sores in the first place.

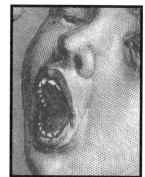

Brew yourself a nice cup of tea, and after you've enjoyed it, put the tea bag in your mouth on the canker sore. This should help heal the sore in a matter of days.

You can find myrrh in the Bible and at your local health food store. It comes in several forms, including a tincture. Use a little tincture of myrrh on a cotton ball to dab the canker sore. Don't be surprised if it stings at first. It should quickly feel much better, and the sore should dry up in a few days.

If a canker sore is really bothering you, go to the kitchen shelf where you keep your spices and dig out the tin of dry mustard. Moisten your finger, dab a little of the mustard onto it, and hold it against the sore for five minutes. To get rid of your sore, do this three times a day. I'm not going to lie; it does hurt. However, the canker sore will be gone in two days.

If you'd rather put something sweeter and kinder in your mouth, take a spoonful of blackstrap molasses and keep it on the sore. It tastes good, and the canker sore should soon depart.

Cuts And Scrapes

People often get canker sores after they've had some abrasion in their mouths, when they've bitten their lip or scraped their gums with a toothbrush. Even a small cut presents an opportunity for bacterial infection. If you break the skin in your mouth, take some of the preventive measures outlined above. Also, use a toothbrush with soft bristles and change it often to avoid damaging the mouth's delicate tissues.

Diet Cautions

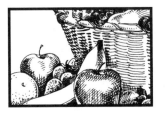

If you routinely get canker sores, increase your intake of foods high in Vitamins B and C, or take daily supplements.

Sugar may be a culprit in causing canker sores. Reduce or eliminate it from your diet if you suffer from canker sores chronically.

Eating an apple a day can keep the doctor at bay and chase away a canker sore, as well. OK, so it might take more than one apple a day. The next time you have a canker sore, try eating an apple after every meal, until the sore is gone. Various substances in the apple promote healing.

LIP BOMB: COLD SORES

Cold sores are caused by the virus herpes simplex. They are contagious and may last three to four weeks.

Keep It From Forming

Taking the amino acid, L-lysine, as a supplement, can help heal a cold sore or prevent one from forming. It's a good preventive measure for those who have a chronic problem, getting more than three cold sores a year. Take 2,000 to 3,000 milligrams a day to keep cold sores away and double the dosage if you feel one coming on. Grandma was a stickler for good nutrition, and you can add lysine to your diet by eating more dairy products, potatoes, and brewer's yeast.

Exposure to sunlight triggers some cold sores, so you should protect your lips with a sunscreen with SPF 15 whenever you go outside.

Taking several acidophilus capsules daily or eating two cups of yogurt with live bacteria a day can help prevent cold sores from forming. The active bacteria seem to boost the body's immune response and may also have anti-viral properties.

Take 400 milligrams of Vitamin C a day to help prevent cold sores. If you feel one coming on, take double the dose. Grandma drank a glass of orange juice every morning, and I never knew her to have a cold sore.

Whenever someone in her family got a cold sore, my grandmother insisted they get a new toothbrush as soon as the sore healed to prevent re-infection. If you feel a cold sore coming on, get rid of your toothbrush immediately. This may keep the sore from actually breaking out. Of course, since cold sores are very contagious, don't come into close physical contact with anybody who has one.

Kitchen Cures

Eat three to four servings of raw vegetables a day for the Vitamin B to facilitate healing and stimulate the immune system. Yogurt will help rebuild friendly bacteria. Take four cloves of fresh garlic a day as a natural antibiotic.

Soothing Salves

Aloe vera was one of Grandma's favorite remedies. She grew her own plant and used it on a wide range of complaints. When somebody in the family felt a cold sore coming on, she would break off a leaf and dab the juice on the area to get rid of it. You can also use a commercial aloe vera gel.

When Grandma could get to the pharmacy, she had Mr. Simpson, our family pharmacist, mix up a solution of spirits of camphor. Dabbing a little on the sore with a cotton ball will help soothe the pain and dry it up.

While at the drugstore, my grandmother would also pick up some petroleum jelly. Placing the jelly on a cold sore can keep it from cracking, bleeding, and spreading.

Apply Vitamin E oil to a cold sore three times a day to get rid of it in a hurry. By the end of the first day, it shouldn't hurt anymore. By the next evening, it should be completely gone.

Make a paste of three tablespoons honey and one tablespoon apple cider vinegar. Place the paste on the sore three times a day to speed healing.

A salve of walnuts and cocoa butter can dry up a cold sore and relieve the pain. Combine a few ground walnuts with a teaspoon of cocoa butter. You'll be rid of the sore in a matter of days.

If you have a cold sore, make yourself a cold drink with plenty of ice. Move the ice on and off your cold sore to reduce pain and inflammation.

Overheard At The Local Bar

The red wine remedy can relieve cold sore pain and dry it up, as well. Put half a teaspoon of red wine in a bowl and leave it there for several hours. When you come back, much of the liquid will have evaporated. Apply what remains to the cold sore for quick pain relief.

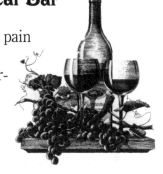

CHOPPER WATCH: DENTURE PROBLEMS

A Perfect Fit

Dentures can be very annoying, even painful, if they are not relined at regular intervals or if they do not fit properly.

Massage gums that are sore from dentures. This increases circulation and decreases sensitivity. However, if you need to use this remedy often, you should have your dentures checked. They probably don't fit properly.

The Old Standby

Grandma's old remedies are just as effective as many new fangled ones. Baking soda is still at the top of the list. It cleans and deodorizes dentures. Stubborn stains should respond to household bleach, but make sure to rinse the dentures thoroughly before wearing them.

Soothing Salt Rinse

Rinsing with warm salty water has a soothing effect since the salt draws fluid from the tissues and reduces swelling. The mixture should be eight ounces of warm water to one and a half tablespoons salt.

BEATING BACK BACTERIA: PLAQUE

Grandma had her own way of removing dental plaque. She recommended drinking two cups of black tea daily to inhibit the growth of plaque forming bacteria from decaying foods. Recently, this was proven by researchers from Washington University.

THE ROOT OF THE PROBLEM: TOOTHACHE

Dab Away The Pain

Grandmother's remedy for a toothache was to place a small amount of oil of cloves on the affected tooth. There is a chemical in cloves that soothes the nerve and eliminates the pain transmissions to the brain for a period of time. The time will differ from person to person. Usually the pain can be controlled with one application on a cotton swab for up to two to three hours.

Put a few grains of cayenne pepper on the aching tooth and gum. This will hurt more at first, but it will go away soon, and so will your toothache.

If you have an aloe vera plant, cut a piece of a leaf and squeeze the gel directly on the aching tooth. Repeat as needed until the pain is gone.

A Sweet Side Effect

Here is a remedy that made us feel better in two different ways: vanilla extract. She would put some vanilla extract on a cotton ball and rub it on the sore area. The alcohol content of the vanilla will help to numb the toothache. And taking the vanilla out of the cupboard always made Grandma feel like baking.

Two Ways To Use Tea

Soak a white washcloth in a cup of prepared chamomile tea. Wring out the tea, and place the warm washcloth on the outside of your mouth (your cheek or jaw) in the area where your toothache is. Dip the washcloth in the tea again whenever it begins to cool. The chamomile should draw out the pain after a few applications.

Drinking sage tea can help relieve toothache pain. Make a stronger cup of tea than you usually would, and hold the tea in your mouth for about thirty seconds before you swallow. The pain should dissipate by the time you've drained your cup of tea.

Not For Teetotalers

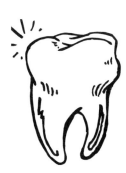

One toothache remedy that should be reserved for adults only is whiskey. Soak a cotton ball in the beverage, and rub it on your troubling tooth and gum. The anesthetic qualities of the whiskey should hold you over until you can get to your dentist. Again, although the remedy doesn't call for you to drink the whiskey, it is still not recommended for children.

Grandpa's Yarrow Escape

Whenever Grandpa would get a toothache, Grandma would make him a yarrow poultice. She would steep a heaping teaspoon of yarrow in just a few ounces of boiling water. She would let it sit for a minute while she cut the cheesecloth. Then, she would strain the liquid and put the saturated herb in the cheesecloth. She'd give it to my Grandfather who would hold it on his aching tooth until he fell asleep in his favorite chair.

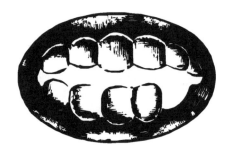

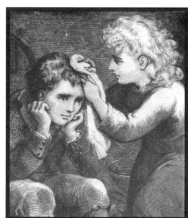

Chapter 5

THINGS THAT GO BUMP

THE BUZZ FACTOR: BEE STINGS

In the United States, the majority of problem bee stings come from honey bees and yellow jackets. If you are allergic and get stung, seek medical care immediately. The stinger should be carefully removed with tweezers as soon as possible.

It can be tricky to get a stinger out without releasing the poison into the body. Grandma was the expert bee-stinger remover around her house. She would pass a wet bar of soap over the area, and it seemed to come right out.

Take The Sting Out Of The Sting

Apply ammonia on a cotton ball to a bee sting for quick relief.

Since ancient times, mud or clay packs have been used to alleviate the discomfort of stings of all kinds. The cooling sensation and the mild drawing action help relieve the pain.

Ice packs or a few ice cubes placed in a piece of cheesecloth will dull the pain of a sting.

Tears And Celery

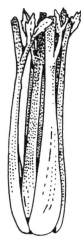

More than once when I was young, I ran into an angry hornet. If you've ever met a hornet, you know that their stings are one of the worst. They tend to cause more pain and discomfort than any other type of insect sting. Grandma would dry my tears, then she would have me chew a small piece of celery stalk and place the pasty mixture of saliva and celery on the site of the sting. Try this in an emergency. You will be pleasantly surprised that the throbbing and the pain will subside in a short period of time. Two or three applications will probably be needed to bring the bite under control.

Swell Ideas For Reducing Swelling

Crush a charcoal tablet and place on a cotton ball. Attach to the sting with a Band-Aid to reduce pain and swelling.

A slice of cold onion placed on a bee sting or insect bite will stop pain and swelling.

Grandpa always had a chaw of tobacco with him, even though he tried to hide it from Grandma. It proved handy when any of us kids got stung by a bee. Moistened tobacco applied to a bee sting can help reduce pain and swelling.

Aspirin is one of the most common home remedies for a variety of complaints, even bee stings. Make into a paste with water and apply to reduce pain and swelling. Don't try this remedy if you're allergic to aspirin.

A paste made from baking soda can be used effectively once the stinger has been removed. A paste made from meat tenderizer, pineapple, or papaya will also work.

PUTTING THE PRESSURE ON: BLEEDING

For a serious cut or gash, try placing powdered cayenne pepper or powdered kelp on the injury to stop the bleeding. Native Americans have used this treatment for hundreds of years. Apply the cayenne (also called capsaicin) to the wound and place a dressing over it. Within a few minutes, the bleeding should have stopped completely. The cayenne increases peripheral circulation, bringing additional blood clotting agents to the area.

YOU SHOULD SEE THE OTHER GUY: CUTS AND SCRAPES

Cleaned And Dressed

One of the best treatments to cause fast blood coagulation is to place an "herbal bandage" on the cut using the herb yarrow. Both the leaves and the flower tips can be pressed into the wound before it is washed and bandaged.

Whenever you need to stop the bleeding from a small cut, rinse the area thoroughly and dress the wound with any of these substances: papaya pulp, cayenne pepper, a moist tea bag, goldenseal powder, or aloe vera gel.

An Oily Solution To Scarring

Applying vitamin E oil to a cut will help it heal more quickly and prevent scarring. Placing the membrane from inside an eggshell will also keep a scar from forming.

Sweet Ways To Guard Against Infection

One of the best natural remedies to prevent infection of a cut or serious bruise is to use juniper berries. Crush fresh berries to make a paste, apply to the wound in a poultice, and allow to remain for three to four hours.

The next time you get a cut, apply a liberal amount of honey to it to stop the bleeding quickly and prevent infection.

WHEN IT'S MUGGY AND BUGGY: OTHER INSECT BITES

Most insect bites are harmless, however some cause some discomfort and may be more serious, requiring professional medical attention. These include tick bites that can transmit Lyme disease or Rocky Mountain spotted fever, and mosquitoes that may carry malaria.

Just Say No

Avoid alcoholic beverages if you will be in an area with mosquitoes. Alcohol causes the blood to come closer to the surface, making you a tempting target.

Say Ahhh

Rub brewer's yeast and garlic into the affected area to help relieve discomfort. A slice of raw potato may also help.

Meat tenderizer can be used to relieve pain and itching. Dissolve a quarter to a half teaspoon in a small amount of warm water and apply to the bite.

Be Quick With A Tick

Ticks should be removed as soon as possible using a lighted match and tweezers. Hold the flame near the tick until it withdraws, then use the tweezers to remove it.

CREEPY CRAWLERS BEWARE: PESTICIDE

Finely ground black pepper will rid your home of most crawling insects, including silverfish, ants, roaches and spiders. Grandma used to sprinkle a small amount inside the cabinets in every corner and especially under the sink. We never saw a bug.

RATTLE BATTLE: SNAKEBITE

Since symptoms may vary depending on the toxin released, it is always best to see a physician.

Symptoms may be alleviated by using a poultice of white oak bark and comfrey. Comfrey salve is also very effective on the affected area. Echinacae tea should be drunk three to four times a day for at least three to four days.

TIME FOR THE TWEEZERS: SPLINTERS

Place an ice cube on the splinter for a few seconds before trying to remove it. This will numb the area.

A LOUSY WAY TO LOSE WEIGHT: TAPEWORM

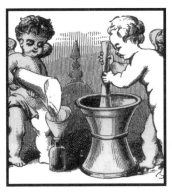

A remedy that has been around for hundreds and hundreds of years is to use pomegranate seeds to chase the worms away. Just dry the seeds from nine pomegranates in direct sunlight or gradually in a low-temperature oven overnight. The seeds are then crushed into a powder with a mortar and pestle or hammer. Use one tablespoon of the powder in a six ounce glass of unsweetened pineapple juice three times a day, preferably on an empty stomach.

WATCH THEM WIGGLE: WORMS

There are many varieties of worms that can infest the human body. They may cause loss of appetite, diarrhea, nausea, anemia, colon disorders and rectal itching. They are more common in children because of their poor bathroom habits.

What's In A Name?

The herb wormwood is recommended in capsule form. Black walnut extract is also excellent. Chaparral tea consumed three times a day on an empty stomach will also have excellent results.

Chapter 6

OH, MY ACHING...

FEELING CREAKY: ARTHRITIS

In basic terms, arthritis is the inflammation of a joint. There are many types of arthritis, which may occur in any of the joints in the body. Most cases of arthritis are characterized by pain, swelling, and deterioration of the joint.

A tried and true remedy that works, depending on the severity of the arthritic condition, is to rub Ben-Gay on the affected area. This provides heat and soothes the discomfort.

Feeling Under The Weather

While grandmother really didn't know the cause of her joint aches and pains, she somehow knew that changes in the weather and certain foods seemed to irritate the problem. When she felt a flair up, she avoided tomatoes, potatoes that had any green on them, eggplant, red and green bell peppers (yellow was OK), all varieties of chili peppers, and paprika. What Grandma didn't know is that many of these vegetables fall into a category known as the nightshade family and may contain the chemical solanine. Solanine has been known to cause inflammation in animal studies.

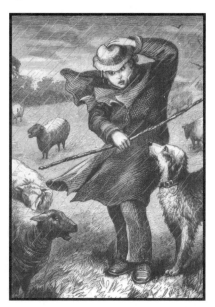

Some Dos And Don'ts

Take one tablespoon of salmon oil daily at lunch and supper. Avoid milk since Vitamin D may irritate sore joints. Also, avoid red meats and paprika. Drink only distilled water.

Work It Out

Exercise is good for everybody. One of the prime benefits is increasing flexibility and keeping the joints in good working order. Nothing could be more important for the arthritis-sufferer. Also, strengthening the muscles will take stress off the joints. The exercise need not be strenuous. Walking and swimming are great options. Grandma started her day with a walk through the woods. "It gets you going!" she always said.

Try Some Alphabet Soup

It's amazing what good nutrition can do for you. Taking supplements of vitamins C, B6, and E can help relieve arthritis pain. The minerals calcium, zinc, magnesium, and beta-carotene may also be helpful. Whenever you add supplements to your daily routine, you should consult your doctor for the safe, effective dosage.

Some Hot Tips

Applying heat to aching joints makes good common sense. It certainly did to Grandma. She recommended a hot bath, heating pad, hot water bottle, or simply wrapping up in a snugly quilt.

Heat some coarse salt in a frying pan and make it into a poultice. Applying it to the affected parts of the body should draw out toxins and speed relief.

If you have arthritis, getting out of bed in the morning can be very difficult. Even if you don't have arthritis, you may feel stiff when you first wake up. Keeping your muscles warm during the night can prevent morning stiffness. Some people pile up the covers, use an electric blanket, a hot water bottle, or heating pad to keep warm. However, getting your night's rest in a sleeping bag seems to work the best, since it keeps in your body's own heat and distributes it more evenly. Just because you're using a sleeping bag doesn't mean you have to sack out on the floor, that would only make your stiffness worse. Stay in your own bed to get the benefit of this cure.

Take These Remedies With A Grain Of Salt

Folk wisdom says that carrying a raw potato in your pocket will draw the toxins out of the body and heal arthritic joints. Change the potato every couple of days as it darkens and dries up. If you prefer a more direct potato cure, cut up two cups unpeeled potatoes and boil them slowly in five quarts water until the liquid is reduced by half. Once the water is cool enough not to burn the skin, immerse a washcloth in the potato water and place it on the sore joints. Keep repeating this process until the pain lessens.

Grandma advised friends with arthritis to wear a copper bracelet. It's not specially scientific, but my grandmother swore by it. The worst part is that your wrist may turn green, but there won't be any other side-effects.

Folk wisdom tells us that rubbing joints once a week with peanut oil will prevent arthritis.

According to traditional German folk wisdom, a cat will carry away your arthritis pain. Have your pet tabby sit on the affected joint to cure your arthritis. Even if it doesn't work, you'll have spent some quality time snuggling with your cat.

The Root Of The Problem

Native American healers treated arthritis with a mixture of mashed yucca root and water. Look for yucca root tablets or capsules at your local health food store and follow the instructions on the package.

Fish And Vinegar

Fish oil has given some people relief from arthritis symptoms. You can take it in capsule form, one a day for the average person. If you don't like to take supplements, try eating more fish. Be sure to choose varieties that are high in fat, such as salmon, tuna, and mackerel, among others.

When your symptoms flare up, try apple cider vinegar. You can either drink it or put it in your bath. If taking internally, add the vinegar and twice as much honey to a glass of warm water. Soak in hot water with one cup vinegar and one cup Epsom salts.

Fruit Juice For Your Joints

Eating cherries is a delicious way to fight arthritis pain. You can choose any variety you like. You can buy fresh, frozen, or canned. Drink at least one glass of cherry juice a day, the all-natural variety without sugar added that you can buy at your local health food store. Some traditional wisdom says you should drink plenty of cherry juice for four days in a row and then go four days without drinking any. Keep repeating this cycle to cure your arthritis. Other people benefit from eating regular amounts of cherries and drinking a glass of cherry juice every day. Experiment to see what works best for you.

White grape juice is reputed to absorb the bodily toxins that cause arthritis. Drink a glass at breakfast and another before dinner every day.

Try a tropical treat to reduce arthritis inflammation and pain. Drink a glass of fresh pineapple juice, twice a day, one after lunch and the other after dinner. If you don't have a juicer and can't find fresh pineapple juice at your local grocery or health food store, you can also used canned or bottled juice, as long as it is all-natural, without additives or preservatives.

• Oh. My Aching... •

Fresh Advice From Grandma's Garden

My grandmother planted an extensive garden every year, with vegetables, herbs, and flowers. There was nothing better than having a summer dinner at Grandma's house with plenty of homegrown food. I remember how fresh those string beans tasted. I could eat them every day. If you have arthritis, you should make it a point to eat string beans as often as possible. The combination of vitamins, minerals, and other compounds in this vegetable seem to correct the arthritic condition.

Grandma also had a flower garden that was the envy of her friends. Lucky for them, she liked to share—especially when it came to helping treat arthritis pain. Try this one yourself. As they begin to wilt, take the petals of three or four of the flowers and put them in a hot bath. You'll feel well-pampered, and your joints will thank you.

Rubbing You The Right Way

Rubbing painful joints with a soothing liniment or salve can bring down swelling and soothe discomfort. Try any one of these arthritis rubs: a mixture of a half teaspoon eucalyptus oil and two tablespoons olive oil; ginger juice, made from squeezing grated fresh ginger root through a cheesecloth, combined with the same amount of sesame oil; and aloe vera gel, which can also be taken internally to treat arthritis. Gently massage the sore areas with any of these salves.

Rub the affected area with oil of bay. Grandmother used to take a few of the leaves and heat them in a small amount of pure olive oil using low heat for approximately thirty minutes. The oil never cooks if the heat is kept low. If the oil starts smoking, add a small amount of Canola oil. After allowing them to simmer for the thirty minutes strain off the oil and use the oil on the affected areas.

Grandma's Cornsilk Curative

To treat arthritis, my grandmother would walk out to her garden, pick a few ears of corn, and bring them back to her kitchen. She would shuck the corn and pick out the silk, putting about a handful into a cup of hot water about ten minutes. When the tea had finished steeping, she'd give a warm cupful of the brew to the arthritis sufferer. If you're not lucky enough to have a garden like Grandma, you can also use corn silk extract or dried corn silk which you can find at your local health food store.

Herbal Relief

A number of herbs are effective in reducing the pain of arthritis. Experiment with rosemary, nettles, basil and sage. You should take several cups of these herbal brews a day, either alone or in combination with one another.

The herb alfalfa relives some symptoms of arthritis. Take at least three to four capsules per day. You may also take alfalfa in the form of a tea three to four times a day to treat pain.

Brew a tea of fresh parsley by steeping one cup of the leaves in one quart boiling water for fifteen minutes. Strain and refrigerate. Take a half cup before your morning meal and another before the evening meal. Take a dose whenever your arthritis pain becomes severe.

Remedies From Around The World

In traditional Romanian healing, celery is cooked in milk and eaten to treat arthritis. Celery does appear to have certain properties that lessen the symptoms of arthritis. You can also eat raw celery or juice the vegetable and drink it. Try to get some celery every day to lessen the effects of arthritis.

Seaweed is a regular part of the Japanese diet, and the incidence of arthritis in Japan is significantly lower than it is in the United States. If the idea of eating a lot of sushi doesn't appeal to you, take powdered kelp diluted with water instead. You can find kelp at most health food stores. Take a half teaspoon of the powder in a cup of warm water every evening before going to bed. You can also take kelp pills if you prefer.

Healing Miss Betsy

Arthritis doesn't seem to run in our family, and Grandma was spry and energetic her whole life. But her best friend and next door neighbor, Miss Betsy, suffered something terribly from rheumatism. Grandma would go next door whenever Miss Betsy's joints were really bothering her to whip up her cabbage cure. She'd take one of the cabbages from her garden and steam a few leaves in Miss Betsy's kitchen. My grandmother would then rub some olive oil into Miss Betsy's knees and ankles where she had her arthritis and when the cabbage leaves were just cool enough she'd lay them on top. Miss Betsy would cover her legs with a towel to keep the heat in, and they'd repeat the process about an hour later. Miss Betsy always said that if it weren't for Grandma and her cabbages she would have ended up bed-ridden, instead of being able to get up, play with her grandchildren and take care of her house.

A Little Smelly But Worth A Try

When you have an attack of arthritis pain, rub a fresh clove of garlic over the sore area. Taking two garlic pills or capsules each day can also help prevent symptoms.

Make a poultice by stirring three tablespoons of horseradish into a half cup boiled milk. Place the mixture in a piece of cloth and apply it to the affected joint. Leave the poultice on the sore area until it cools. You should feel much better.

No Pain, No Gain

Cayenne pepper cures many ailments, and it seems to have long-term benefits in treating arthritis pain. Take one or two cayenne capsules, three or four times a day, every day. The bad news is that you will probably notice an increase in pain at first. The good news is that quickly afterwards the pain will begin to decrease, and in the long run, you'll feel much relief from painful joints. Because this remedy does contribute to pain at first, you should only undertake this treatment with the help of your doctor.

Grin And Bear It

Here's the best news you've heard all day. . . having sex can help combat arthritis pain! Sexual stimulation releases cortisone in the body which counteracts pain.

The Caffeine Cure

Some of the most delicious coffee in the world comes from Puerto Rico, and it seems like no coincidence that coffee is the main ingredient in the traditional Puerto Rican remedy for arthritis. Whatever variety of coffee you prefer, make yourself a hot cup first thing in the morning and add the juice of one lime. It's purported to greatly reduce pain and swelling.

LIFT FROM THE KNEES: BACK PAIN

Relaxation Therapy

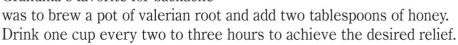

The herb valerian root taken in capsule form or prepared as a tea tend to relive the discomfort through the relaxation of the muscles. Grandma's favorite for backache was to brew a pot of valerian root and add two tablespoons of honey. Drink one cup every two to three hours to achieve the desired relief.

Whenever anyone in her family had a bad back, Grandma recommended a soak in a hot tub with Epsom salts, not too long, about twenty minutes. Chiropractors and physical therapists often prescribe the same thing. Alternating hot and cold may also help, taking a hot bath or shower one day and applying an icepack to the sore area intermittently throughout the day the next.

A warm poultice can help relax muscles and speed relief from back pain. Try using flaxseeds the next time your back is tired and sore. Soak a cup of the seeds overnight. When you're ready to make your poultice, boil the seeds and tie them up in a piece of cloth when they have cooled just enough not to burn the skin.

The Straight And Yarrow

Taking a daily dosage of yarrow tea can help heal a problem back. Brew the tea from a teaspoon of dried yarrow and a cup of boiling water. After it steeps for ten minutes, strain and drink. Take a cup before each meal and one just before going to bed.

Leave On The Leaves

My grandmother's cabbage cure for arthritis is also helpful for treating back pain. Steam a few leaves until they're slightly wilted, about ten minutes. Rub the sore area with olive oil and place the cabbage leaves on top of it as soon as they are cool enough for you to stand. Be careful not to burn your skin. Put a towel over the area to retain the warmth. Leave it on for an hour and then repeat the whole process.

Healing Hands

A massage can bring relief from back pain for at least several hours, especially if you use Grandma's homemade rubbing liniment. Mix a pint of rubbing alcohol with three ounces wintergreen oil and two tablespoons powdered white willow bark. Allow to sit in the sun for two hours and strain. Warm slightly and massage the affected area.

Make a liniment from one pint rubbing alcohol, two ounces of wintergreen and a dozen aspirin. Massage into sore muscles. Don't try this remedy if you're allergic to aspirin.

Rocking Away Back Pain

When my grandparents were first married, Grandpa made a rocking chair for Grandma. Grandpa was quite a carpenter, and it was a beautiful piece of furniture, fashioned out of walnut, with wide armrests and a curved back. Grandma would sit in the chair in the evening and work on her crocheting. Whenever Grandpa's back was acting up on him, she'd make him sit in the old rocker, and by the time he was ready to go to bed, the pain would have almost disappeared. It wasn't just a fluke, either. It seems that rocking can help increase circulation and block pain signals in the lower back. As an added bonus, it's soothing and relaxing.

Ideas From The East

Traditional Asian medicine recommends soaking your feet to ease a bad back. Leave your feet in warm water for twenty to thirty minutes.

Asian healers prescribe black beans to heal back pain. Get a bag of dried black beans at the grocery store and prepare them according to the instructions on the package, but without salt. Eat a couple of tablespoons of the beans every day for a month. Don't store the beans in the refrigerator for longer than three or four days. Make fresh batches as needed.

A Spoonful Of Relief

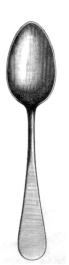

To promote overall healing, take cod liver oil, which is rich in Vitamins A and D. One tablespoon, three times a day will help aide in the healing process.

White willow bark contains the active ingredient salacin, an aspirin-like compound, effective for treating pain, including that of the back. It is usually taken in tincture form, one teaspoon three times per day for severe back pain.

TENNIS ANYONE?: BURSITIS

Bursitis is an inflammation of the bursae, small sacs filled with fluid found in the joints, bones, muscles and tendons. They cushion the bones against friction during movement. Numerous injuries of the bursae can occur, the most frequent from calcium deposits and increased stress on a particular area, such as the elbow with resulting "tennis elbow."

• Oh. My Aching... •
Grandma's Bursitis Plant

My grandmother came from Europe in the early 1900s. She didn't have much, just two bags and a plant she carried under her arm. When she came to Ellis Island, she was not allowed to bring her plant into the country. That well-travelled plant was the herb arnica. My grandfather had a serious problem with recurrent pain in both shoulders from doing heavy farm work for many years. The only thing that ever relieved his pain was a salve made from arnica. Although her plant didn't survive the journey, her remedy did: Prepare a salve by placing two tablespoons of powdered arnica in just enough olive oil to make a loose paste. This needs to be applied to the affected area twice per day and left on for twenty minutes. Cover it with a washcloth slightly dampened with water as hot as you can comfortably stand.

The Jekyll And Hyde Of Exercise

Exercising the affected joint is the most effective way to relieve discomfort. Ice packs will help reduce any swelling, which will speed the healing process.

Bursitis can be caused by overdoing exercise, pushing the body past its current fitness level. Exercise can also be the cure. The trick is to re-establish a full range of motion for sore muscles. You might try lifting weights, preferably under the supervision of a trainer or physical therapist. More simply, swing your arms in large circles in both direction, or stretch arms above your head by walking fingers up a wall. Remember that pain is a message. If a particular movement hurts, don't push it.

A Sleeping Cure For Shoulder Pain

Whenever someone in the family had bursitis or some other shoulder problem, Grandma would want to know how they had been sleeping, whether they laid on the arm with it above their head. Nine times out of ten, they did. She'd tell them to be careful of how they sleep, keeping the arm out of the way, and they'd usually feel better in a matter of days.

A SWELL JOINT: GOUT

Gout is related to uric acid levels in the blood, urine and tissues. The acid tends to crystallize in certain joints, especially the large toe. Ninety percent of the cases occur in men. Uric acid is derived from certain foods, and a low-purine diet is recommended. Foods high in purines are meat, anchovies, asparagus, herring and sardines.

Drier Is Better

If you have gout, avoid alcohol, even small amounts. Alcohol interferes with proper liver functioning, allowing more of the toxin that causes gout to build up in the body. Drinking alcohol also causes dehydration which can aggravate gout.

Teetotalers' Treatments

Hyssop tea gives relief from gout, especially if combined with juniper.

Certain herbal teas help clean out the toxins that cause gout. Yarrow, dandelion, and celery seed work especially well. You can use them individually or in combination with one another. Take three or four cups a day to keep gout away.

An old country cure for gout is a daily dose of corncob tea. Cut the kernels off several ears of fresh corn, put the cobs in a stew pot and cover liberally with water. Let the mixture simmer for an hour, remove the cobs, and retain the liquid. Store the corncob tea in a sealed jar in the refrigerator. After each meal, take a cup of the tea. Do this every day until the pain is gone.

Juicy Tidbits

An age-old cure for gout is to drink eight ounces of black cherry juice every day. This remedy may also affect some arthritic conditions.

To relieve the painful symptoms of gout, follow a mostly-strawberry diet. For several days, try to eat little besides strawberries. Certain sub-stances in strawberries seem to relieve inflamma-tion, which will reduce the discomfort caused by this ailment.

Garlic Lovers' Take Note

The traditional Russian remedy for gout is getting more fresh garlic into the system. Try to eat at least two cloves a day. You can mince the garlic and eat it in a salad or sprinkled over a meal. You can also swallow it with a glass of water, like a pill. This garlicky cure will keep away the gout, as well as vampires.

BE STILL MY ACHING HEAD: HEADACHES

Most headaches are caused by stress, diseases related to the eyes and sinuses, high fevers, or allergies to perfumes, after shave lotions and other products. Poor alignment of the cervical vertebrae may also contribute.

A number of herbs made into teas cab be used effectively to reduce a headache's severity or totally relieve it. These include goldenseal, hyssop, lobelia, mint and burdock root.

Grandma's 30-Minute Migraine Mend

One day my Aunt Beatrice was suffering from a severe headache, the kind that would probably be called a migraine today. To relieve her pain, grandma peeled several bananas. Although Aunt Beatrice said she wasn't hungry, Grandma kept right on peeling. To our surprise, she put aside the fruit and made a poultice of the skins. She placed the poultice on 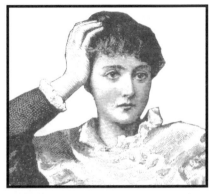 my Aunt's forehead and back of her neck. The headache was gone in about thirty minutes. And we all enjoyed the banana bread after supper.

Brushing Away Headache Pain

Whenever somebody in the family got a headache, Grandma would take out her favorite silver-handled hairbrush and gently brush their hair, away from the temples and down the back of the head. She would hum a little tune, just under her breath, and it wasn't too long before the headache was gone and you felt much better. It appears that brushing helps increase blood flow to the area which speeds relief.

Forehead—Aches

For this old world cure, all you need is a potato and a bandanna or towel. Slice the potato and stick it under the bandanna tied tightly around your forehead. The combination of moisture and pressure eases the pain.

Whenever my grandmother got a headache, she would dip a rag in vinegar and tie it around her forehead until the pain disappeared.

• *Oh. My Aching...* •

She'd usually be feeling better in an hour or two.

Rub your forehead and temples with a lemon peel, with the rind against your skin. Secure it in place with a bandanna and leave it there until the headache is gone.

Cold Cures

Apply an ice pack to the back of the neck or forehead for headache relief.

Try the cold water cure for a headache. Fill your bath tub with cold water, just enough to cover your feet, and walk back and forth for a few minutes, no more than five. The rest of your body should be covered and warm. Once your feet begin to feel warm in the cold water, get out, dry off your feet, and get into bed. Snuggle down into your covers, rest, and your headache should disappear pretty quickly.

Advice From Our Forefathers

Colonial Americans treated headaches with a mixture of one teaspoon honey and a half teaspoon garlic juice.

Another sage idea: grate some fresh horseradish and make a poultice out of it. Apply it to the back of your neck to relieve headache pain.

Pressing Possibilities

By rubbing the roof of your mouth with your thumb you can interfere with the nerves' ability to carry pain signals. Press into a certain spot for five minutes and then move to another place on the roof of your mouth. You should feel relief almost immediately.

Traditional Chinese healers prescribe acupressure to relieve headache pain. Take turns rubbing the second joint of each thumb, first the right and then the left, for two minutes each. Repeat five times on each thumb. If you use your favorite scented lotion, you can imagine you're getting a hand massage at the manicurist.

Aspirin Alternatives

Aspirin will cure a headache, but it upsets some people's stomachs. Almonds contain the same active ingredient, so try eating a couple dozen almonds in place of taking aspirin. It might not work as quickly, but it tastes much, much better!

Strawberries contain a compound that is similar to the active ingredient in aspirin. If you'd rather not take over-the-counter medication to get rid of your headache, try eating a few strawberries instead.

Vaporize A Headache

Grandma kept a big jar of Vick's vapor rub on her bedside table. When she had a headache at night, she'd put a dab on each temple to open up her sinuses and relieve pressure and pain. You don't have to wait for bedtime. Use this remedy any time a headache has you down. Also, if you prefer, you can use peppermint oil instead of Vick's. If it's not comfortable to apply the oil directly to the skin, take a hot bath, using a few drops in the water, and breathe deeply. Oil of rosemary also helps get rid of a headache. Put a few drops on your temples and under your nose.

Breathing in vinegar vapors can help relieve a headache. Mix a cup of apple cider vinegar and a cup of water and bring to a boil. When the mixture begins to steam, turn the heat down as far as it will go, place a towel over your head, and breathe in the vapors, for about ten minutes.

The Key Is To Relax

Getting a massage is a great way to relax. Since many headaches are caused by muscle tension, getting your neck and shoulders rubbed can ease the pain of a headache. It's a great excuse to get your partner to give you a back rub!

Angelica is effective as a pain killer and can be used to cure a headache. Brew a tea by adding a half teaspoon of the herb to a cup of boiling water. Steep and drink it down. It will soothe and calm you.

Try a compress of basil and witch hazel to relieve headache pain. Heat a teaspoon of basil in a cup of water, and add two tablespoons of witch hazel. Once it's cool enough to touch your skin, dip a cloth in the mixture and lay it across your forehead. It's even more effective if you lie down and relax while it's working.

Vitamin And Mineral Supplements

Taking a magnesium supplement can help relieve and prevent headaches. Up to 400 milligrams is considered a safe daily dosage, but you should check with your doctor before starting any supplement.

Studies have shown that vitamin C effects constricted blood vessels. If you have chronic headaches, try taking a Vitamin C supplement. Your doctor can advise you on a safe and effective dosage.

Pressure To Relieve Pressure

According to traditional Chinese healers, it is important to get more blood circulating in your upper body, and less to your head, in order to knock out a headache. Swing your arms around wildly. This should lessen the pressure in your head and give you a break from your pain.

TAMING HORSES: LEG CRAMPS

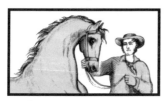

Leg cramps may be caused by a number of circulatory problems. Inefficient blood flow in the lower extremities is common as you age. One of the most frequent complaints is called intermittent claudication.

Get The Kinks Out Of Your Diet

There are a number of vitamins that may help relieve leg cramps. Vitamin B-6 has had good results, but check with your doctor for dosage recommendations before you try these.

Vitamin E benefits the circulatory system in many ways, and it seems to have positive effects in relieving night foot and leg cramps. Take up to 400 IU of vitamin E daily. For higher doses, you should consult a physician.

People who take diuretics may suffer from leg cramps. If this is the case, add bananas to your diet to make sure you get enough potassium. A banana or two each day should replace the potassium you are losing.

Since this is sometimes caused by a deficiency of calcium and magnesium it would be wise to consume foods that are high in these minerals such as dark green leafy vegetables and whole grains.

You may be able to reduce the occurrences of leg cramps by changing your eating habits. Leg cramps my be an indication of a calcium deficiency, so be sure to include plenty of greens in your diet. Eat them raw or steamed to get the most benefits from the vegetable's nutrients. Also, try eating less sugar, white flour and fatty meats for a week. See if you notice a difference.

Stretch It Out

If you feel a muscle about to tighten up, take a moment and stretch it. You can also stretch a muscle that's already cramping, but the technique is more effective if you use it to ward off a cramp.

Improving your blood circulation can prevent muscle cramps. When you wake up in the morning, and when you go to bed at night, lie on your back and raise your legs above your body. Lean your legs against a wall, the end of the bed, etc., and keep them elevated for about ten minutes. Twice a day should do the trick.

Putting Discomfort To Bed

Grandma was always after us kids to keep our feet warm. She was convinced that walking around on a cold floor could bring on leg cramps. If you have a problem with spasms in the legs and feet, try wearing a pair of warm, wool socks to bed.

Leg cramps that occur at night can be relieved with this sweet and sour remedy. In half a glass of warm water, mix one teaspoon of honey with one teaspoon of apple cider vinegar and one tablespoon of calcium lactate. You should be feeling better in less than half an hour.

Grandma's Silver Lining

When I was little, I remember neighbors coming by to ask Grandma's advice for different ailments. Lucky for them, she made house calls, and lucky for me, she took me along. When one of her neighbors, Miss Betsy, complained of being woken up in the middle

of the night by leg cramps, Grandma went right to Miss Betsy's silver drawer and pulled out a spoon. She said to keep it next to
her bed, so the next time she felt her leg seizing up, Miss Betsy
could put the spoon right on the cramp. It must have worked
great, because two days later, Miss Betsy came to the house
with a big smile on her face and one of her famous apple
pies. If you are going to try this remedy, your spoon
needn't be silver, stainless steel will do.

Wash Away The Pain

Here's a soothing tea that can wash away leg cramps.
Some say if you drink one cup of red raspberry leaf tea
twice a day—in the morning and in the evening—you
may say good-bye to leg cramps for good.

Pinch Away The Pain

Try this remedy in a pinch. Some say it works almost instantly.
When you first feel a leg cramp, pinch the skin between your upper
lip and your nose with your thumb and index finger. Put your fingers
on either side of the "divet" and keep pinching this point for about
twenty seconds and the cramps should disappear. This is especially
effective for people who get leg cramps while swimming.

BLINDED BY THE LIGHT: MIGRAINE

This severe throbbing headache, normally centered behind an eye
or at the back of the head, may last for ten to fifteen hours before
subsiding.

The herbs feverfew and ginko have had excellent success in treating migraines. Feverfew reduces or eliminates the pain, while
gingko biloba increases circulation.

Grandma's Cabbage Compress

The next time you get a migraine, try my Grandmother's cabbage leaf compress. Our Aunt Beatrice was a migraine sufferer, and she would always turn to one of Grandma's remedies for relief. I remember this remedy was called upon quite a bit.

Soften a few leaves in boiling water—just dip the leaves in until they get soft. When they cool off a bit, place a leaf or two on your forehead and a leaf or two on the nape of your neck. Grandma would keep the cabbage in place by wrapping bandannas around Beatrice's head and neck. Once the leaves are secure, relax and let the cabbage do its work. Grandma claimed that the cabbage would draw out the pain, so when she threw the leaves away, she said she was throwing the pain away.

Pressure Is The Point

Acupressure can be helpful for many ailments. Try this technique the next time you feel a migraine coming on. With your right thumb, apply pressure to your left palm. Keep the pressure firm—especially if you're feeling tenderness in the area—for five minutes, then switch hands and repeat.

Look Good, Feel Better

Some people find that sitting under a hair dryer relieves migraine tension. The heat and hum of the dryer can be very relaxing and very effective.

Hold The Cold Cuts

If you are prone to migraines, keep a jar of very strong mustard on hand. When you feel the pain coming on, open the jar and breath the fumes deeply. Many people have found this helps relieve their discomfort.

Try the double Spanish onion remedy. Boil two onions, one is for eating and one is for mashing into a poultice and placing on your forehead.

LOOSEN UP: MUSCLE STIFFNESS

This is a common complaint. Certainly anybody who has done intensive manual labor or has worked out too vigorously at the gym has had stiff muscles or a backache. One of the best herbs to relieve muscle stiffness is chamomile. To prepare a massage oil, place three cups fresh chamomile flowers in a pint bottle and add enough extra virgin olive oil to cover them. Place the mixture in direct sunlight for two to three weeks, then refrigerate until you need to use it. The oil may be warmed to a comfortable temperature.

Soothing Soaks

My grandmother kept Epsom salts in the cupboard where she stored the ingredients for her home remedies. It was one of the products to which she turned most. Nothing is more relaxing than settling into a hot bath with Epsom salts. The salts, which are mostly magnesium, greatly ease tension and also draw out the fluids which often collect in tired muscles.

Here are two bathtub suggestions that are effective for helping a charley horse. Make a relaxing ginger bath by preparing a strong ginger tea. Boil two teaspoons of ginger powder or fresh ginger root in two cups of boiling water. When the water turns yellowish in color, the ginger tea is ready to be added to your bath. Soak for a relaxing twenty to thirty minutes to relieve muscle stiffness. Ginger is also excellent for the circulation.

• *Oh. My Aching...* •

The other charley horse bath is one you've probably heard of. That's because it usually does the trick. Pour three cups of Epsom salt in a warm bath. Soak for twenty to thirty minutes to ease the pain.

Make Lemonade

For muscle stiffness (especially for a charley horse) try this citrus solution. In a blender, place two small oranges cut into pieces, three small lemons cut up and one small grapefruit cut into pieces. Be sure to use the whole fruit, skin and all. Add one teaspoon of cream of tartar and blend. Place the citrus blend in a covered jar or bottle and store in the refrigerator. Twice a day—when you wake up and right before you go to bed—take two tablespoons of the citrus blend with two tablespoons of water.

Homemade Muscle Rubs

For an old Hungarian remedy for sore muscles, mix cayenne pepper with vegetable oil and rub into the affected area. Use a quarter to a half teaspoon pepper to one cup warm vegetable or baby oil. Cayenne pepper contains the active ingredient capsaicin that blocks the transmission of pain signals.

Make ginger juice by grating the ginger and squeezing it through cheesecloth. Measure the juice and add an equal part sesame oil. Massage the mixture onto your sore muscles as needed.

Hot And Cold Running Cures

Both heat and cold have their places in treating sore muscles. If you strain a muscle while working or exercising, apply an ice pack as soon as possible, no more than twenty minutes after the injury. This will help reduce swelling and pain. Taking a hot shower helps relax muscles which relieves pain. Direct the shower stream to the sore area. If you place a washcloth on the spot, it will retain heat and increase the relaxing effect.

The Farmers' Muscle Salve

My grandmother was always on the lookout for new remedies. One day while she was at the drugstore, she saw several elderly farmers ask Mr. Simpson, the pharmacist for the same thing, one right after the other. They all wanted wintergreen rubbing alcohol and a bottle of aspirin. Mr. Simpson explained to Grandma that they dissolved the aspirin in the alcohol to treat sore muscles and joints. A number of his customers swore by it. Grandma added the two items to her list, and it's been one of her favorite remedies for muscle ache ever since. Of course, she never gave it to anyone who was allergic to aspirin.

Apple cider vinegar is another sore muscle solution. Slowly boil two cups of apple cider vinegar and one tablespoon of cayenne pepper in a glass saucepan. Put it in a jar or bottle and use it on your sore muscles.

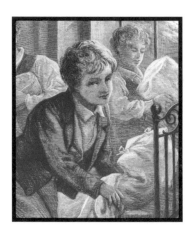

Chapter 7

IN THE OUTHOUSE

THE DRY IDEA: BED-WETTING

This condition is usually found in young boys who have not mastered the control of their bladder. It is rarely found in girls. In adults the problem tends to surface in the later years as incontinence or loss of bladder control.

Tinkle, Tinkle Little Star

Grandma used to help children with this problem by teaching them muscle control. She would have the child stop and start the stream of urine. Children should attempt to do this at least six to eight times whenever they urinate.

Wake Them For Bathroom Breaks

To cure bed-wetting problems, wake up children a few hours after they've gone to bed, some time before midnight, for a trip to the bathroom. Children tend to wet the bed when they are in the deepest sleep, near the beginning of the sleep cycle. After a few weeks of doing this, children should be able to wake themselves up when they need to go to the bathroom.

Putting Them To Bed

Don't allow the child with bedwetting problems to have any liquids at least two hours before bedtime. This may mean no liquids at supper until the problem is resolved.

Give your child a cup of corn silk tea just before bedtime to help keep the bedclothes dry. You can make the tea by adding ten to fifteen drops of corn silk to a cup of boiling water. Be careful to let the tea cool before giving it to your child to avoid a burned tongue.

A classic bed-wetting remedy is to give your child a teaspoon of raw honey before sending them off to bed. As always, it is best to use locally produced honey. In the morning, you should find dry sheets and a well-rested child.

Some Natural Choices

No one seems to know why, but cinnamon bark has had great success in preventing bed-wetting. Have your child chew on a piece of the bark throughout the day. The child should have no problem making it through the night.

The next time you're at the local health food store, look for bone meal tablets. Giving your child one tablet after every meal should help stop bed-wetting. As your child becomes more and more able to wake up to use the bathroom, decrease the dosage.

A Tranquil Solution

My grandmother insisted on quiet time for everybody before going to bed, children and adults alike. She'd turn the radio off, and we'd all talk quietly, growing more and more sleepy. When I was young, she'd tuck me into bed and read a soothing bedtime story. As it turns out, my Grandma's tranquil bedtime hour is also a great idea if your child has trouble wetting the bed. Studies show that watching television, especially shows that are scary, violent or anxiety-producing, contribute to bed-wetting. If your child is having trouble waking up to go to the bathroom, try Grandma's solution. Declare quiet time for everybody. You'll be doing less laundry in a matter of no time.

Not Just Kid Stuff

To treat incontinence in adults, take a tea made from the herb uva ursi. Brew the tea from a tablespoon of the leaves in a cup of boiling water. Let it stand for five minutes before straining. Seal the tea tightly in a jar to store. Take a tablespoon before each meal. If you continue the treatment for six weeks, you end up with dry sheets at night. This cure has never been recommended for children who wet the bed.

FEELING THE BURN:
BLADDER INFECTIONS (Cystitis)

Cystitis is an inflammation of the bladder usually caused by a bacterial infection. It tends to be more prevalent in women because of the proximity of the anus to the vagina, which facilitates bacterial transmission. Escherichia coli is the cause of most urinary tract infections.

Proper hygiene habits can prevent bladder infections. After going to the bathroom, women should wipe themselves from front to back. Don't share soap, towels, or other bathroom items with family members or guests.

Drink Me A River

One of Grandma's preventive measures for bladder infections was to make sure that she drank at least eight glasses of water daily. She knew this helped but really didn't understand the reason; by keeping the bladder well hydrated, it reduces the buildup of residues which are the breeding ground for bacteria. Note: Make one or two of these glasses of fluid cranberry juice. It will be even more effective.

Then Drink Some More

Another of Grandmother's cures for bladder infections was to have you mix one teaspoon of baking soda in eight ounces of water and drink the mixture everyday for two to three days. This may also relieve any burning sensations. A caution should be noted in that this mixture should never be taken after a meal due to the fact that if you consume a large meal it may be dangerous to over bloat your stomach and cause a possible rupture.

While the thought of drinking garlic juice may not appeal to you, Grandma recommends squeezing the juice of a whole garlic into a glass of cranberry juice. In two to three days the problem will usually clear up.

Take two capsules of acidophilus, three times daily. Drink plenty of liquids, including eight ounces of cranberry juice. Always use pure juice from a health food store that has no added sugar. Bacteria has difficulty multiplying in an acidic medium.

And Then There's Tea

A tea made from the herb uva ursi (or taking two capsules a day) has been known for hundreds of years to relieve and speed up the healing of kidney and bladder infections. The extract may also be used by following the directions on the bottle.

To remedy bladder infections and heal kidney maladies, brew a tea from the dark green leaves of the prince's pine plant, also called pipsissewa, which grows wild in hardwood forests. You can find the herb at your local health food store. It is safe to take several times a week for extended lengths of time to treat chronic urinary tract problems.

Native American healers used cornsilk tea to treat bladder infections and other urinary tract problems. To make the tea, steep the silk from one ear of corn in three cups boiling water for five minutes. Seal tightly in a jar and store on your cupboard shelf. Take several cups a day whenever you get a bladder infection. If corn is not in season, you can also use cornsilk extract, found at most health food stores.

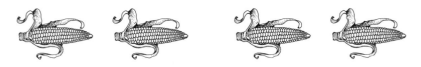

C If You Feel Better

Take 1,000 milligrams of Vitamin C a day to acidify urine and clear up a bladder infection. Research suggests that taking this dosage on an ongoing basis to prevent infection is safe. Larger doses than this should only be taken for specific periods of time. Consult your doctor.

The Cultured Cure

Some women treat a bladder infection by eating large amounts of yogurt, three or four cups a day. While this may or may not cure an infection, it will definitely help prevent one. The friendly bacteria in yogurt, acidophilus, helps prevent bad bacteria from growing. If you're prone to bladder infections, eat more yogurt with live cultures or take acidophilus capsules to help ward them off.

Baking Soda Bliss

To relieve the burning and discomfort that accompany a bladder infection, soak in a hot tub with baking soda added to the water. Stay in the bath at least thirty minutes.

COLON CARE: COLITIS

Colitis is the inflammation of the colonic mucous membrane which creates small pouch-like areas, causing cramps and diarrhea. If it becomes very severe, ulcerations may occur.

Cleansing the colon is one of the best remedies for colitis. Consuming a diet high in fiber with an adequate amount of oat bran and steamed or raw vegetables. Hyssop is an effective cleansing herb. Drink at least eight glasses of water a day.

HOW TO BE A REGULAR JOE OR JANE: CONSTIPATION

This occurs when waste material moves too slowly through the large intestines. It is caused by a low fiber diet, lack of moisture, or both. A number of drugs may also cause constipation, especially those with a high iron content.

The Java Jolt

For many people a cup of regular coffee seems to relieve constipation. Caffeine activates the peristaltic action of the intestines.

Diet Additions

Herbs commonly used to treat constipation include hyssop, flax seed and psyllium seed. Prunes act as a natural laxative. Over-the-counter preparations can be overused and may reduce good bacteria in the intestinal tract.

Eat a high fiber diet, with at least three to four servings of fruits and vegetables and two to three servings of whole grains a day. This diet, along with adequate liquids, will alleviate the problem in a day or two.

Eat a baked apple for supper and another for breakfast the next morning. This works almost every time and is a lot more pleasant than an enema.

Believe it or not, a little Mexican food can help you get back on track. That's because eating an avocado mixture, very much like guacamole, can ease constipation. Mash up a ripe avocado and some chopped onion, a little lemon juice, and a dash of cumin. Enjoy your fiesta!

Persimmons may also help relieve constipation. Eat one a day when they're in season.

Soybeans Do The Trick

For a natural cure for constipation, boil two to three tablespoons of black soybeans in two quarts of water for ten to fifteen minutes. Simmer and reduce until there is only one quart left. The mixture can be seasoned as desired. Consume one glass three times a day until the problem is alleviated.

Friends and Enemas

When it came to constipation, Grandma said an enema bag was your best friend. She also swore by two tablespoons of mineral oil before bedtime. Lucky for us kids, she gave us a choice. So unless we were doubled over with discomfort, we would always take the mineral oil.

Grandma's Constitutional—A Constipation Cure

Grandma was always busy, working in her garden, canning vegetables, baking bread, visiting with company, but she made time every day for a long walk. Her morning constitutional, she called it. Exercise has many health benefits, including preventing and relieving constipation. You don't have to do wind sprints either. A mild stroll for fifteen minutes every day should help keep you regular.

Natural Laxatives

The natural, water-soluble fiber psyllium aids in moving food through the digestive tract. You can get psyllium seeds at your local health food store. Use them on other foods or simply take a teaspoon a day, chew, and swallow with a glass of water.

Flaxseeds have properties similar to psyllium. Make a laxative "goop," with flaxseeds ground in a coffee grinder mixed with apples, oranges, and grapefruit processed in a blender. Take three table-spoons of ground flaxseed with an equal amount of fruit everyday.

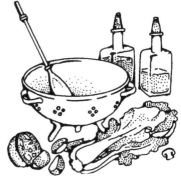

Escarole, spinach, okra, and Spanish onions are natural laxatives. Try eating escarole or spinach raw in salads. If you prefer, you can boil the escarole and drink the juice. Gumbo is a delicious way to get more okra in your diet. Eat roasted Spanish onions, preferably in the evening before going to bed. If you start the day by eating two small, fresh beets, you should have no problems with your digestive tract functioning.

Another of nature's most perfect foods is brewer's yeast. It is highly nutritious, a concentrated source of many vitamins and miner-als. It also helps ease constipation. Many people take brewer's yeast in combination with wheat germ. The optimal dosage for most peo-ple seems to be a teaspoon of brewer's yeast and another of wheat germ. But start out slowly to give your body a chance to adjust to the change in your diet.

Grandma's "Regular" Smoothie

Grandma always had a little rhubarb growing in her garden for pies and constipation remedies. Place three chopped rhubarb stalks (without the leaves, they're poisonous), one cup apple juice, a quarter peeled lemon, and one teaspoon honey in a blender, and process until smooth.

Salty, But Sweet Relief

Sauerkraut juice helps relieve constipation. If you don't want to make your own, like Grandma did, you can get it canned and drain the juice. You won't want to use this remedy too often, since it's very salty and excessive amounts of salt can be harmful.

Herbs That Make Scents—And A Little Pressure

There are several herbs that treat constipation. Sacred bark usually starts to work eight hours after it's taken. Senna is used in a number of over-the-counter laxatives. Goldenseal and bayberry are also helpful.

Certain scents seem to have positive effects on a constipation problem. Draw yourself a warm bath and add twelve or so drops of rosa gallica. Enjoy your bath for at least fifteen minutes and repeat three times a week.

Traditional Chinese medicine recommends acupressure to get rid of constipation. Rub the spot between your bottom lip and chin. Keep doing this until you begin to feel relief. It shouldn't take more than fifteen minutes.

Bulk Up On Fiber

Bulk up on fiber, which helps keep the digestive tract functioning regularly, by adding raw bran to your favorite cereal. You should give your body time to adjust to the higher level of fiber in your diet by starting out slowly, with a teaspoon or so, and working up to a tablespoon or two.

A Spoonful Of Relief

Olive oil is a wonderful food. It is a staple of fine cooking, and it tastes great. This delicious oil has many health benefits, as well. It helps lower cholesterol and helps the digestive tract function normally. You can take olive oil as a natural laxative, one tablespoon in the morning and another after dinner.

Grandma's huge jar of blackstrap molasses came in handy when someone in her family was constipated. An hour before lunch, she would have them take a teaspoon of the molasses in about a half cup of water. It seemed to clear the problem right up.

Rise And Shine

Start your morning with a fresh glass of juice. If you prefer fruit juice, drink orange or grapefruit. Any number of vegetable juices will help relieve constipation, including cucumber, celery, cabbage, and beet. Carrot juice seems to be especially helpful. Taking a tablespoon of aloe vera juice, available at the local health food store, twice a day, once in the morning and once before bed, is a fine remedy for constipation.

To help yourself have a bowel movement in the morning, drink a cup of warm water with the juice of half a lemon in it before having anything to eat. You can also drink prune juice, or eat prunes, apples, figs, or papaya for breakfast to stimulate the bowels.

Cure constipation with cloves. Before going to bed, fill a mug with half a cup of boiling water and add six or so cloves. Let it set overnight and drink the water in the morning. You'll be on your way to more regular bowel movements.

A Sunny Cure For Constipation

Grandma liked to snack on sunflower seeds, the ones she harvested from her garden. She kept a large bowl of them on the kitchen counter and ate them raw, without salt. Sometimes, she'd add a handful to a salad she would serve to the rest of the family. Sunflower seeds are just plain good for you, and Grandma swore her daily snack helped keep her regular.

BULKING UP: DIARRHEA

Characterized by frequent, loose, watery stools, and abdominal cramping, diarrhea can be caused by drugs, bacterial infections, spoiled foods and a number of diseases. It is associated with dehydration and subsequent mineral loss. Medications should not be administered for at least 36 hours to give the body a chance to rid itself of the toxin that is causing the problem.

Combine one teaspoon finely chopped raw garlic with one teaspoon of honey. Take this remedy three times a day, about two hours after each meal.

Grandma's Juicy Secrets

Grandma learned from her mother to always keep blackberry juice in the ice box for these occasions. She had us drink four ounces of the juice and we'd be feeling "right and steady" in no time. Blackberries are a tasty and effective treatment for diarrhea. You can take the blackberries in many different forms: frozen, fresh, or even blackberry wine. Try this recipe to make a gallon of blackberry wine: Crush four quarts of wild blackberries, add a gallon of boiling water, and let stand 24 hours. Add three pounds sugar and strain. When it starts bubbling, it's time to bottle it.

• In The Outhouse •

Bananas add fiber and potassium to your system which helps relieve diarrhea. This is one remedy you won't have trouble getting your children to take!

Another of grandma's cures for diarrhea was to grate up one large apple and allow it to stand at room temperature for three to four hours until it turned brown before eating it. When the pectin oxidizes it tends to produce a chemical that is found in many over-the-counter remedies for diarrhea.

Dairy Does It

The good bacteria in yogurt and acidophilus capsules helps balance bad bacteria in the intestines and remedies diarrhea.

Combine two tablespoons cottage cheese and two teaspoons sour cream. Take the mixture three or more times a day, depending on the severity of the problem, until the diarrhea clears up.

Cure For Cramps

Use ginger tea to alleviate pain or cramping. Chamomile tea may be helpful in slowing the diarrhea or stopping it completely.

Ice packs can take away the discomfort associated with diarrhea. Put one on the middle of your back and another on your lower back. Leave the ice on for ten minutes and then take it off for ten minutes. Keep going this way as long as it feels good.

Bland, But Beneficial

You should follow a bland diet, with plenty of complex carbohydrates, while you have diarrhea. Try eating mostly rice, potatoes, bananas, toast, and apples.

· *In The Outhouse* ·

It's always a good idea to add brown rice, something of a wonder food, to your diet. It's low in fat, high in complex carbohydrates and fiber, and an excellent source of B vitamins. Following a diet high in fiber can help keep the digestive tract functioning smoothly, preventing both diarrhea and constipation. If you do come down with a bout of diarrhea, you can also use the rice water to cure the problem. Boil a half cup brown rice in six cups of water for thirty minutes. Strain the rice and retain the water. Sweeten it with honey and drink one cup every other hour. Do not drink any other liquids until the diarrhea clears up.

From the ancient Greeks to Grandma, barley water has long been used to cure diarrhea. Put a quarter cup of barley in six cups of water, boiling until the liquid is reduced by half. Strain out the barley, and keep both it and the water. Drink the barley water as a tea, using lemon and honey to flavor it if you like. It will help keep you hydrated as it returns your bodily systems to normal. You should also eat the barley, which is good for you anyway.

Restoring Friendly Bacteria

Drink one to two glasses a day of any of these beverages: buttermilk, sauerkraut juice, or kefir, a product you can find in your local health food store. These substances help restore friendly bacteria to the system that prevent the bad bacteria that cause diarrhea. You can also get these helpful bacteria by eating pickled vegetables or raw sauerkraut.

Keep It In The Cupboard

Vinegar has definite anti-bacterial properties. If you come down with a bad case of diarrhea, take a tablespoon of apple cider vinegar in a glass of water before each meal, following a bland diet until the condition clears. The vinegar should help kill the bacteria that are causing the problem.

Take one teaspoon cornstarch in a glass of water. This cure is fast-acting, but it doesn't work for everyone. If you don't see results in three hours, start another treatment.

Look for carob powder at your local health food store and keep it on hand to treat diarrhea. When you're sick, take a tablespoon in a glass of warm water and drink it down. Use this remedy before each meal.

The spices cinnamon, allspice, and cloves can be used to relieve diarrhea. One variation on this theme involves putting a little of the spice in warm milk. Try a pinch of all-spice in a cup of warm milk; two pinches of cinnamon in warm milk; or two pinches of cinnamon with a pinch of powdered cloves in warm milk. Another easy way to take cinnamon is on a piece of apple. Cinnamon may be even more effective and fast-acting when used in combination with cayenne pepper. Brew a tea by adding a quarter teaspoon of cinnamon and an eighth teaspoon of cayenne pepper to two cups of water. Reduce the heat and allow to cook for twenty minutes. Let it cool and drink half a cup every hour.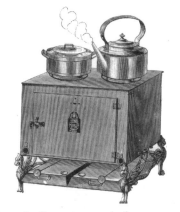

Activated charcoal will absorb most anything. It's used in hospital emergency rooms to treat cases of poisoning. You can find activated charcoal capsules or tablets at your local health food store. Take a couple of the capsules or pills to absorb the bacteria or other agents that are causing your diarrhea.

Give The Runs The Raspberry

There were wild raspberry brambles in the woods behind Grandma's house. In the summer, my friends and I would go with her to pick them, eating two for each one we put into our buckets. Grandma would also pick some of the raspberry leaves. When we got back to the house, Grandma would make the raspberries into the most wonderful desserts—cobbler, pie, and homemade ice cream. She would dry the leaves and store them in the cupboard with the other ingredients for her home remedies. Whenever I got a bad case of diarrhea, she would fix me a cup of raspberry leaf tea, and I would soon feel better. She put two ounces of the leaves in two cups of water and cooked it over low heat for twenty-five minutes. She'd strain out the leaves, let it cool, and give me cups of it to drink throughout the day. Sometimes, Grandma would also cook a cinnamon stick in it because I liked the taste, but that part is completely optional.

Lousy Timing—A Tip For Travelers

There's nothing worse than getting sick while on vacation. Unfortunately, diarrhea often strikes when we drink water that contains bacteria our bodies aren't used to. This is a standard remedy relied upon by international travelers and recommended by various nations' health services. Pour a glass of orange juice, or any other fruit juice, and mix it with half a teaspoon of honey and a pinch of salt. Fill another glass with purified water. Drink from one glass and then the other. Keep alternating beverages until all the liquid has been consumed. You should feel better by the next morning.

TEAR REPAIR: FISSURES

Anal fissures are small tears that occur around the rectum and may cause discomfort or even pain. They are mainly caused by excessive straining during bowel movements. Inadequate consumption of liquids may contribute to the problem, causing the stool to be too solid. Constipation is a common problem associated with these fissures.

One of the best preventatives is a small amount of Vaseline regularly applied to the affected area. Aloe vera is also effective when used in the same way. A warm sitz bath, sitting in a small amount of water with your knees raised, will help relax muscles and provide relief from anal fissures.

LETTING OFF STEAM: FLATULENCE

This ailment is usually caused by foods, such as beans, that contain a complex sugar difficult for the body to break down. These sugars often ferment which produces gas. A number of other foods are also guilty, including cabbage, broccoli, and corn.

No Beans About It

Grandma had a great way to cook beans "without the rumbles." Place a teaspoon of fennel seed in the water that the beans soak in. The fennel seed neutralizes the complex sugar and eliminate the gas problem.

Before And After

If you are going to eat food that typically produces gas, try a tea made from fennel. Drink a cup with your meal and it should eliminate the problem.

• In The Outhouse •

Activated charcoal is naturally absorbent and can relieve excess gas. Take a capsule or two with a meal when eating foods that normally make you gassy. It should help lessen the problem.

If you have a chronic problem with gas, take a tablespoon of aloe vera gel or juice after each meal. It should help keep the rumbling and bubbling under control.

Papaya, a sweet and delicious fruit, contains enzymes that help the body digest food more easily. If you can't find fresh papaya in your grocery store, look for chewable papaya pills at the health food store. The good news is that they taste great, like candy. Eat four papaya pills after a meal whenever you think you might get heartburn.

Milk—For Better Or Worse

For people who are lactose intolerant, eating dairy products can cause stomach discomfort and gas. Try any of the over-the-counter remedies that supply lactase, the enzyme necessary to break down the sugar found in dairy products.

The bacteria found in yogurt will also help break down milk sugars. You can eat more yogurt with live cultures or take acidophilus capsules. This friendly bacteria also contributes to the healthy functioning of the intestines.

Help From Herbs

There are a number of herbal teas that can help relieve flatulence. Try peppermint, parsley, anise, ginger, and chamomile.

Take a cup of bay leaf tea to soothe the stomach and get rid of gas. To brew the tea, add a half teaspoon of the herb to a cup of boiling water. Allow the mixture to steep, strain, and drink it slowly to settle the stomach.

149

• In The Outhouse •

Relieving The Pressure

Regular exercise is good for the digestive system. Take a walk or bike ride to help rid the body of excess gas.

If you have gas pains, apply a hot compress to your abdomen for relief.

A simple mixture of anisette liqueur and a cup of warm water will soothe the stomach and help the body expel excess gas.

The Onion Sandwich Cure

Some of my grandmother's remedies are not for the faint of heart. Grandma had a stomach of iron. She loved raw garlic and onions fresh out of the garden. On the odd occasions that she had a problem with gas, she would fix herself a raw onion sandwich and eat it with gusto. For her, it was a treat that also did the trick in getting rid of the gas. If onions don't agree with you, definitely don't try this remedy, or you're likely to end up with gas and heartburn.

A ROYAL PAIN: HEMORRHOIDS

Hemorrhoids are veins that have become swollen and enlarged. They are normally found around the anus and frequently protrude out of the rectum. They may occur as a result of childbirth, obesity, straining during bowel movements, or even prolonged periods of sitting in one spot. Symptoms include itching and occasional bleeding.

Vitamin C is the cure for many of the things that ail us, including hemorrhoids. The only difference is that you take it on the outside, rather than the inside. Take a cool bath with powdered ascorbic acid dissolved in it. Soak for at least fifteen minutes. It's most effective if you repeat the treatment a couple of times a day. It should help speed healing.

Soothing Compresses

Try a poultice saturated with a warm solution of any of these effective herbs: parsley, hyssop, buckthorn leaves, stone root and grape vine leaves.

My grandmother used a simple poultice of cottage cheese to treat hemorrhoids. Place the cottage cheese in a cheesecloth or handkerchief and apply to the painful area. To maintain effectiveness, you should change the poultice three times a day.

Apply a poultice of white bread dipped in egg white to the site of the hemorrhoids. This should take away the pain and bring down the swelling.

You Want Me To Put It Where?

A small raw potato (peeled) or a peeled clove of garlic inserted as a suppository may provided relief.

Create a cranberry suppository by grinding up a quarter cup of cranberries in a blender and placing them in a cheesecloth. Insert the suppository into the rectum and replace after an hour, using fresh cheese cloth. After the second time, you should feel a reduction in pain and itching.

A Good Witch

Grandma swore by an age old cure to relieve the symptoms: witch hazel. Place extracts of this plant on a warm washrag and cover the affected area. The witch hazel will soothe and relieve the problem for hours.

Soothe The Itching

Zinc oxide will soothe hemorrhoid itching. You can purchase it in over-the-counter preparations, such as Desitin which is intended for diaper rash. It will coat the affected area and keep you from scratching.

Grandma didn't have Noxzema, but some home healers recommend it to relieve hemorrhoid suffering. Apply it with a tissue to help reduce itching.

To relieve hemorrhoid pain and itching, eat a large leek, preferably boiled, every day in the afternoon or at supper time.

Reduce The Pain And Swelling

There are a number of natural ingredients you can apply with a moist cotton ball to hemorrhoids to relieve the discomfort and reduce swelling. Try vitamin E or wheat germ oil; a mixture of a half teaspoon dry mustard and a tablespoon of honey; papaya or lemon juice.

Applying ice to hemorrhoids can help reduce swelling and relieve pain. By the time the ice melts, you should be feeling better.

Take a long soak in a warm tub to lessen hemorrhoid discomfort. The heat causes the muscles to relax which reduces pain.

In One End To Soothe The Other

Take one to two teaspoons of linseed oil daily as a stool softener.

For an internal remedy, take a teaspoon of aloe vera juice after each meal until the hemorrhoids are healed.

LET 'ER RIP: LAXATIVE

Dates are one of the best natural laxatives. A few dates eaten every day will keep you regular. Try consuming six to seven dates followed by a glass of warm filtered water twice a day.

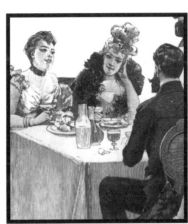

Chapter 8

HERE'S THE SKINNY

ARE YOU GONNA EAT THAT?: APPETITE

B-complex vitamins stimulate the appetite center in the brain. To increase your appetite, take a half teaspoon of brewer's yeast, an excellent source of these vitamins, daily. If you are on a weight control program you should try and regulate your intake of Vitamin B and not overdo them with supplements.

ALL DAMMED UP: WATER RETENTION

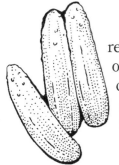

One of the best diuretics to reduce excess water retention is watermelon or cucumber tea. Many melons work as a diuretic since they contain a chemical called cucurbocitrin. This chemical increases the ability of the cells to release fluids to the kidney's for release.

BATHROOM SCALE BLOWOUT: WEIGHT CONTROL

Grandma's Flapjack Diet

Believe it or not, Grandma believed in eating buckwheat pancakes to lose weight. This is one great way to take off the pounds and enjoy yourself at the same time. Two pancakes for breakfast will keep you from getting hungry for at least five hours and will reduce your desire for heavy meals the balance of the day. It's a great appetite suppresser and much more fun to eat than celery and carrots.

Fill Up On Liquids

There are many herbal teas that you can buy at the health food store that are quite good for curbing the appetite: raspberry leaves, fennel seeds, yerba mate (this contains caffeine), cleavers and horehound. Use one tea bag, or if you prefer, one teaspoon of the dried herb. Drink one cup of tea a half hour before each meal and another cup before you go to bed.

To help you feel full, drink tomato juice ten or fifteen minutes before you eat.

Sweets Relief

To help curb your desire for sweets, slowly drink three ounces of pure grape juice diluted with one ounce of water a half hour before each meal and before you go to bed. Take several minutes to drink and be sure the grape juice has no sugar added and no additives or preservatives. Your cravings for desserts should start to disappear, making it easier for you to make healthy food choices.

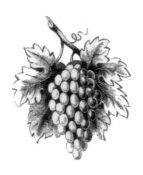

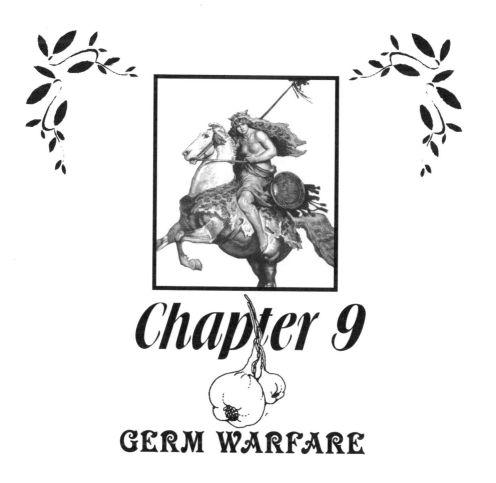

Chapter 9

GERM WARFARE

Historically, severe infections were cause for amputation, because treatments were not effective and the disease progressed to a life-threatening stage. Grandma had a remedy for infections that were very unusual and worked almost every time. She would take young alfalfa sprouts, grind them up and add two cups water and one cup unsweetened grapefruit juice. Alfalfa is a rich source of chlorophyll which was used by physicians in the 1940s to treat patients who had post surgical infections. The mixture may be placed in a juicer or blender and you should consume four ounces twice each day. She also recommended a diet of fresh vegetables and whole grains while you are sick.

A FUNGUS AMONG US: CANDIDACIES

Candidacies is a yeast-like fungus commonly found in the genital tract, mouth (thrush), throat, vagina (vaginitis) and intestine. It is characterized by itching and a white cheesy discharge. Symptoms vary depending on the part of the body involved and may include: canker sores, joint pain, sore throat, heartburn, numbness, arthritis, cough and hyperactivity.

Avoid all wheat products and reduce sugar and carbohydrate intake, including fresh fruit which is high in fructose. You should also avoid vinegar. Consume yogurt to help rebuild friendly bacteria.

TURNING GREEN: FUNGAL INFECTIONS

Yeast or mold, common funguses, can affect many areas of the body, including the vagina, mouth, nails and skin. A reddish patch

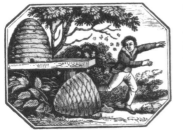

anywhere on the body may indicate a fungal infection. Fungal infections often appear when the immune system has become weakened.

One of grandma's favorite remedies for fungal infections was honey. Apply it to the affected area for thirty minutes. Replace with fresh crushed garlic and leave for another half hour.

ALL FIRED UP: INFLAMMATION

Inflammation occurs when the body reacts to an infection or trauma. It may also be caused by some disease processes such as arthritis or by straining a muscle.

• Germ Warfare •

Certain herbs have historically been used to reduce inflammation, including goldenseal, red clover, pau d'arco and echinacea. They should be taken in capsule form for the best results.

A SPOTTY REPUTATION: MEASLES

This viral infection affects the respiratory tract and is accompanied by skin rash and itching. It is highly contagious, easily spread by coughing and sneezing. Look for white spots in the throat as one of the first symptoms.

Taking a tea made from catnip or an extract of lobelia every four to five hours may help. Try garlic enemas to lower the associated fever.

GETTING YOUR LUMPS: MUMPS

This serious infectious disease is caused by a virus and usually strikes in childhood. It is contagious two to six days after the onset of symptoms. The infection causes the swelling of one or both of the parotid glands in the sides of the neck. Mumps can cause sterility in both of the sexes.

A tea from the herb echinacea reduces swelling. Drink a cup three to four times a day. You may reduce pain by using lobelia extract, a half teaspoon every three to four hours. Be sure to increase fluid intake during the course of the illness.

159

ALL STRESSED OUT: SHINGLES

Blister Balm

Treat sores with a mixture of eighty percent pure honey and twenty percent Vaseline. It should help ease the pain. Honey is the only food on which bacteria will not grow; it has been used since the ancient Egyptians to heal leg ulcers, eczema, and many skin problems.

For a soothing remedy, apply a paste of baking soda and water to the affected area. It should bring relief pretty quickly.

Make a healing tea of buckbean to relieve the discomfort of shingles. Boil two cups of water and add one ounce of dried buckbean leaves. Let the tea steep for approximately ten minutes and place in a jar. Before each meal, take four tablespoonfuls of the tea. Within a short time, you should be feeling better.

The Bees Knees

There are several bee products that can be helpful in easing the pain and promote healing. Spread raw honey on the lesions several times each day until the pain goes away and you can see the lesions healing. Bee propolis is another product that can do wonders for those suffering form shingles. Be sure to get the liquid form, available at most health food stores. Cover the lesions with the liquid by using a soft brush (try a clean, unused makeup brush). Do this several times throughout the day, and you should see a big difference.

When You Can't Scratch

If you experience itching, apply fresh leek juice to the affected areas. Your itching should stop right away.

Pierce a vitamin E capsule and spread the oil on the blisters. This will help stop the itch and will promote healing. Repeat throughout the day.

Like many skin ailments, shingles can be helped by aloe vera gel. If you have a plant around, cut off a part of a leaf and squeeze the gel onto your skin. The itching should disappear almost instantly.

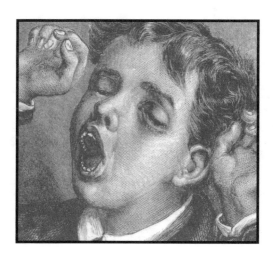

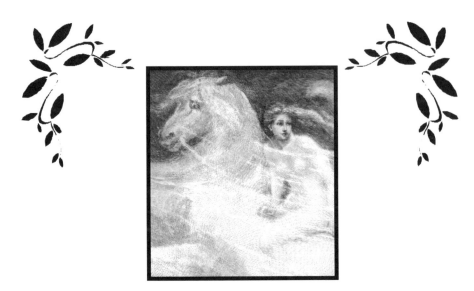

Chapter 10

IN WITH THE GOOD AIR, OUT WITH THE BAD

WAITING TO INHALE: ASTHMA

This serious, even life threatening, lung condition is caused by an inflammation of the small bronchioles which creates shortness of breath. It may be triggered by a reaction to allergens such as dust, pollens and smog. Mucous may also build up in the airway causing more discomfort.

Avoiding An Attack

Food allergies can bring on an asthma attack. Common trouble-makers are seafood, especially deep-water fish, since they contain histamines which can trigger breathing problems. Food preservatives can also irritate asthma, including MSG (monosodium glutamate) and sulfites. Try avoiding these foods to see if they may be contributing to your breathing difficulties.

Dust is a common allergen. To reduce the level of dust in your home, place cheesecloth over heating ducts. Vacuum cleaners also put out a great deal of dust into the air. You can place cheesecloth, a single layer, over the exhaust vent, or buy products specifically designed to reduce the amount of dust given off by your vacuum cleaner.

If you come into contact with an excessive amount of pollen, wash off immediately. This will help prevent or lessen an attack.

Garden Variety Cures

Siberian ginseng has been used for hundreds of years to increase vitality and to relieve shortness of breath.

Take a tincture of mullein orally to clear congestion and relieve asthma symptoms. You can find it in most health food stores.

When you hear the word "licorice," you probably think of strands of chewy candy. However, licorice is an herb used in many traditional remedies. At your local health food or herb store, get a licorice stick. Cut it into smaller pieces, add boiling water, and steep for an entire day and night. Whenever you feel an asthma attack coming on, take a cup of the licorice brew.

Some people swear by cherry bark tea as an effective remedy for asthma. Take the tea four times a day, before every meal and before going to bed. You should be able to find cherry bark tea at your local health food store.

You can make your own cough drop by putting a drop of eucalyptus oil on a sugar cube. This also seems to help relieve the difficulty in breathing associated with asthma.

Grandma Gets Steamed

Grandma used steam to alleviate the symptoms of many ailments, especially if they were related to the chest or upper respiratory system. She used either a vaporizer or teapot and covered her head with a towel so that she got the full effects of the steam. A little deep breathing, and she always felt better. (She liked the way it made her complexion look, too.)

You can also try putting a pot of sliced, unpeeled potatoes on to boil and inhaling the vapors. The steam should relieve respiratory distress and help you breathe more easily. Steam can cause a serious burn, so be careful not to get too close.

Good To The Last Drop

Recently, studies have shown that asthmatics who drink coffee regularly have fewer attacks than those who don't. Caffeine may have a minor effect on the adrenal glands stimulating them to produce enough hormone to relax the small bronchioles and improve breathing. Grandma recognized this intuitively, and recommended drinking a cup or two every day to alleviate asthma symptoms.

Pour Over The Problem

Try juicing up to prevent or lessen an asthma attack. Look for aloe vera juice at your local health food store and take a small amount, no more than an ounce, after each meal. For healthy lungs, as well as sharp eyesight, drink a mixer of fresh carrot and ginger juice. To make ginger juice, grate some fresh ginger root into a cheesecloth and squeeze. You need about a table-spoon to add to six ounces of the carrot juice. It's a good idea to make this mucous-cleanser a part of your morning routine. You can also take a dose whenever you feel the need for relief. For a super asthma reliever, drink one glass daily of endive, celery, and carrot juice mixed together.

Drink cranberry juice, without sugar added, to treat asthma and other respiratory ailments. Most health food stores sell unsweet-ened cranberry juice. However, if you can't find it in your area, you can make your own by boiling one pound of fresh cranberries in one pint of water until they get very soft. Store in a jar in the refrigera-tor. Take two tablespoons at least thirty minutes before every meal and whenever you feel an asthma attack coming on.

Grandma's Supremely Sunflower Anti-Asthma Syrup

My grandmother always planted a row of sun-flowers in her garden. As a child, my friends and I loved to hide among the stalks that were twice as tall as we were. I always thought Grandma planted them because she thought they were so cheerful, but in fact, she harvested the seeds for us kids to snack on and to make her

Supremely Sunflower Anti-Asthma Syrup. To make your own, boil four cups of sunflower seeds in two quarts of water, reducing the liquid by half. Strain and add one pint of honey. Continue boiling until the mixture becomes syrupy in consistency.

Nutrition Solutions

Some studies suggest that increasing your intake of Vitamin C can help increase lung capacity and decrease bronchial constriction and spasms. Drink more orange juice or take a daily supplement. Consult your doctor for the proper dosage.

To promote healthy lungs and bronchial strength, eat up to six apricots every day. Jerusalem artichokes, eaten every day, can also help nourish the respiratory system.

Tune Up Your Lungs

Music can soothe the savage beast of asthma. Playing a wind instrument, like the flute,
trumpet, clarinet, or harmonica, can strengthen the
lungs, making you less susceptible to any respiratory ailments. It's one of the few treatments for asthma that can actually be called fun.

A Strong And Sweet Asthma Cure

When Grandma's Supremely Sunflower remedy wasn't enough to treat an asthma problem, she would whip up a batch of her honey and garlic cure. She simmered three peeled whole bulbs of garlic in two cups of water until they were soft and the liquid had been reduced by half. She then put the garlic in one of her canning jars. To the garlic water remaining in the pan, she added one cup cider vinegar and a quarter cup honey, boiling the mixture until it reached the consistency of syrup. She added the syrup to the jar containing the garlic, closed it tight, and let it rest overnight. Her recommended dosage was a clove or two of garlic, along with a teaspoon of syrup, every morning before eating anything.

There are several other remedies involving honey that can help relieve asthma symptoms. Combine one teaspoon of grated horse-radish with one teaspoon of honey. Take this treatment every night before going to bed. You can also try the honey-onion cure. In a jar, place two large, raw, sliced onions in two cups of honey. Seal the container and allow the mixture to stand overnight. Wait thirty minutes after each meal and take a half teaspoon. Take a full teaspoon every night before bed.

Meditate On This

Relaxation is perhaps the simplest and cheapest cure. When the bronchioles relax it will shorten an attack or even terminate it completely. Take two to three slow breaths and release all muscle tension.

COUGH IT UP: BRONCHITIS

Bronchitis is caused by the inflammation or obstruction of the breathing tubes (bronchi) that enter the lungs. Symptoms include mucous buildup, fever, coughing and chest pain. In acute cases, it may follow an upper respiratory infection and lead to pneumonia. Because of the inflammation and the resulting difficulty in the exchange of oxygen and carbon dioxide, the heart may work harder, resulting in heart disease.

Use a humidifier. Place boiling water into a shallow pan and breathe in the steam for short periods of time.

SPRING IS IN THE AIR: HAY FEVER

Hay fever effects the mucous membranes of the nose and causes the eyes to tear. Many sufferers have symptoms all year long, especially a runny nose. Some people who have hay fever also suffer from asthma and occasional dermatitis (skin disorders).

Before The Sniffles Start

Hay fever is caused by pollen, so keep your house and car windows closed and the air conditioning on during hay fever season to help reduce pollen levels.

When you get inoculated against a disease, a small amount of inactive pathogen is introduced into your system to help your body build up its own natural defenses. You can do the same thing with hay fever by gradually building up your immunity to granules of bee pollen. Some people are allergic to bee pollen, some quite severely, so start very slowly. Begin with three small granules, and very, very slowly work your way up to a teaspoon a day. 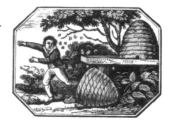 You can take the granules like pills with a glass of water or add them to your food. You can find bee pollen granules at your local health food store or from a beekeeper in your area. Begin the immunization process four months before hay fever season begins.

Supplemental Advice

Take 400IU Vitamin E capsules twice a day. One tablespoon of liquid alfalfa should also be taken twice a day.

Since colds and hay fever have many of the same symptoms, taking Vitamin C may help speed relief for hay fever sufferers. Take 500 to 1,000 milligrams a day until the symptoms clear up. However, you should check with your doctor for the exact dosage.

• *In With The Good Air, Out With The Bad* •

Plan ahead for hay fever season by taking brewer's yeast, according to the recommended dosage on the package. In addition to alleviating some of the worst allergy symptoms, it's also highly nutritious, a great source of various vitamins and minerals.

Cupboard Cures

Consuming two to three tablespoons of locally produced honey seems to eliminate the problem completely. The honey must be produced locally, not just any honey will do.

Take one to two tablespoons of apple cider vinegar a day during hay fever season.

Botannical Brews

As far back as the ancient Egyptians, the herb fenugreek has been used to treat all sorts of respiratory problems, including hay fever. Start drinking a cup of fenugreek tea before every meal at the beginning of spring in March and keep it up for three months. Fenugreek is very powerful medicine and can provide a great deal of relief from congestion and other hay fever symptoms. To make the tea, take four cups cold filtered water and soak nine teaspoons fenugreek seed for six hours. Boil the mixture for three minutes, strain, and drink the tea sweetened with a small amount of honey.

Taking red clover blossoms or horseradish can help increase your resistance to a variety of allergies. Brew a tea from red clover blossoms and take up to four cups a day. You should be able to find red clover blossoms at your local health food store. Mix a quarter teaspoon of horseradish in a glass of juice or hide it in your food, taking a dose every day. Either one of these remedies should strengthen your system and keep you from suffering extreme allergy symptoms.

If you prefer not to take synthetic antihistamines, either over-the-counter preparations or drugs prescribed by a doctor, take nettle to get a natural antihistamine. Take a capsule or two every few hours to stave off sneezing, congestion, irritated eyes, and other hay fever symptoms.

Inhaling Healing

Make yourself a cup of your favorite herbal tea and inhale the vapors to lessen congestion due to hay fever.

Inhaling steam from warm salt water can help open nasal passages. You can also squirt warm salt water directly into your nostrils to clear out a stuffy nose. Dissolve a teaspoon of salt in one cup warm water. Dip with your hand and inhale with one nostril while pinching the other closed.

According to aromatherapists, the scent of lavender or chamomile can relieve hay fever symptoms. You can buy these essential oils at a local health food or herb store. Put a few drops on a hanky and keep it with you. Whenever you feel a sneezing fit coming on, press the handkerchief to your nose to bring the much needed relief.

Quick Relief

My grandmother used to tell anyone who had hay fever or sinus problems to lie down with a cool, wet washcloth over their face. It helps stop sneezing and eye irritation.

During hay fever season, keep honeycomb stocked in your home. Take a small piece and chew on it when you feel an attack coming on.

Keep it in your mouth for ten to fifteen minutes, and of course, spit it out when you're finished. You don't need a ball of wax in your stomach. It should provide relief from hay fever symptoms.

SOMEBODY STOP ME: HICCUPS

A Spoonful Of Sugar

Whenever we would get the hiccups, Grandma would reach for the sugar bowl. Sugar cures hiccups by stimulating the nerve pathways that are transmitting the hiccup reflex signals. Just a spoonful of sugar should do the trick.

Culinary Curatives

To cure hiccups, try a cup of dill leaf tea sipped slowly.

Common wisdom suggests drinking various sorts of juice to cure hiccups, including orange, pineapple and onion.

Grandma considered apple cider vinegar the great cure-all. It was one of her favorite remedies for the hiccups. She would mix a teaspoon of the vinegar in a cup of warm water and have me drink it all down. By the time I finished the last drop, my hiccups would invariably be gone.

Chewing very slowly and thoughtfully can help interrupt the hiccup reflex. Pick something bready and chewy, like a bagel or slightly stale loaf bread. By the time you finish it, the hiccups should be gone.

Take A Deep Breath

Breathe into a paper bag to stop hiccups. Inhaling carbon dioxide appears to return the body back to normal. Concentrating on breathing may also help relax the diaphragm.

Aromatherapists recommend taking deep breaths of sandalwood oil or perfume to ease hiccups.

Pucker Up

Grandma recommended sucking on something sour, like a pickle, to get rid of the hiccups. The shock of a strong taste may jolt the diaphragm's nerves out of their spasms.

Suck on a wedge of lemon with a little Worcestershire sauce on it. This should get rid of your hiccups in a matter of no time.

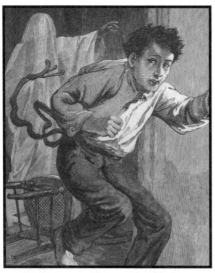

Create A Diversion

Grandma says that if you concentrate hard on something else the hiccups will go away, just like that. Focusing your attention helps the diaphragm relax. Try asking yourself trivia questions. Who was the fifth President of the United States? Name the seven dwarves. Why did the chicken cross the road? Your hiccups should be gone now.

Scaring a person with hiccups or tickling them until they laugh will cure their hiccups. It interferes with the nervous system activity that causes the hiccup reflex.

If you're lucky enough to need to sneeze while you have the hiccups, that will cure it faster than anything. If your body needs prompting, inhale a little black pepper, gently, just enough to make you sneeze. It will blow your hiccups right away!

Put It On Ice

An ice pack is good for many purposes, including breaking the hiccup reflex. There is some disagreement about where the ice pack should go, just below the rib cage or over the belly button. Experiment to see which one works for you and leave it there for five minutes or until the hiccups are gone.

Creative Solutions

Stick your fingers in your ears to cure hiccups and breathe deeply. It temporarily interferes with nerve impulses that control hiccuping.

My cousin Ruth claims that sticking out your tongue will cure the hiccups. She says that Grandma told her about it, but I'm not so sure. Anyway, it does seem to work if you stick your tongue out as far as you possibly can and leave it out there for several minutes.

Traditional Chinese medicine prescribes acupressure to stop hiccuping. Press the center of the sole of your foot until the hiccups are gone.

A Last Resort

If you have a serious case of the hiccups and nothing else will get rid of them, take a hot bath. The heat relaxes your muscles and seems to stop the hiccup reflex when nothing else will.

BROWNBAGGING IT: HYPERVENTILATION

This state of dizziness, heart palpitations, or uncontrollable rapid breathing occurs from rapid intake of air and excessive volumes of oxygen entering the lungs.

Breathe into a paper bag to regulate the amount of oxygen and carbon dioxide that is exchanged. This will reduce the amount of oxygen and increase carbon dioxide, returning both to normal levels.

Stretching will also relieve hyperventilation. Reach your arms as high above your head as possible, stretching as tall as you can, breathing as deeply as possible. This should help slow the rate of breathing and relieve the condition.

EVERY BREATH YOU TAKE: PNEUMONIA

Pneumonia is an inflammation of the lungs usually caused by a bacterial infection, a virus or fungus. The tiny air sacs become inflamed and fill with mucous.

Ginger tea or capsules, as well as goldenseal, have been used to treat pneumonia. However, a physician should be consulted.

HUFFING AND PUFFING: SHORTNESS OF BREATH

Castor oil packs placed on the chest are helpful to assist the bronchioles to open.

RIGHT BETWEEN THE EYES: SINUSITIS

This Inflammation of the nasal sinuses, which often accompanies a severe cold or upper respiratory infection, is caused by bacteria or viral infections. Smoking and the inhalation of irritants also contribute to the problem.

Nasal Knowledge

It is recommended not to use forceful blowing of the nose since this may cause the mucous to go back farther into the sinus cavity. Try sniffing and allowing the mucous to drain to the back of the throat and then expel it. Vaporizers tend to loosen mucous. Adding a small amount of eucalyptus oil to the vaporizer seems to enhance the effect.

A nasal rinse of warm salt water can help clear out mucous and relieve sinus pressure and pain. Mix a half teaspoon of salt with one pint warm water. You can also add a teaspoon of witch hazel if you like. To apply, take a handful and breathe in. You can also use a spray bottle. You should feel the benefits right away. In a couple of days, your sinuses should have completely cleared up.

A Spicy Solution

Have you ever bitten into hot, spicy food and had your eyes water and your nose run? This effect can be annoying when you're eating Mexican food, but if you have sinus problems, it can bring much needed relief. Try taking ten drops of Tabasco sauce in a half cup of water every day. Or you could just eat more salsa and chips. The effect is the same. The active ingredients in the hot food thin out mucous and make it easier to expel it from the body.

If you've ever eaten horseradish, you know how it can clear your sinuses. Use freshly grated horseradish and breath in the vapors. Be very careful—inhale very gently. If you prefer, try eating freshly grated horseradish mixed with lemon juice. Eat one teaspoon an hour before breakfast and an hour before dinner. Many people take this remedy every day and claim long lasting-relief.

To help stifle the sniffles, sprinkle freshly ground pepper on one teaspoon of honey. Swallow, being careful not to inhale the pepper.

From The Health Food Store

This remedy should take about a week to work. Each day, take two parsley pills and two garlic pills every four hours (or, about four times a day).

If you're suffering from a sinus attack, try chewing on honeycomb. Natural honeycomb is available in most health food stores. Use a one-inch square, and chew the waxy gum for about ten minutes after you've already swallowed the honey. The honeycomb can help you breath easier, stop sneezing and you'll probably get a burst of energy as well.

Traditional healers have long used oregano to treat respiratory tract infections and coughs. Make a tea by steeping one to two tea-spoons of the dried herb in a cup of boiling water. It will help loosen mucous, making it easier to blow your nose and cough up the excess phlegm.

The Healing Touch

Massage the face or apply pressure with the fingertips under the cheekbones, to the sides of the nose, and at the bridge of the nose to relieve sinus pain and pressure, as well as congestion. This touching will increase the oxygen supply to the area, which promotes healing.

Running Hot And Cold

Now, here's a hot tip that will promote drainage. When you start feeling symptoms, place hot wet towels on your face. Make the towels as hot as you can stand them, without burning yourself. Keep the towels on the upper part of your face for fifteen minutes, three times a day.

Some people respond to cold rather than heat to treat sinus pain. If a warm compress doesn't work for you, try an ice pack or drink cold water. Since this treatment won't help your body get rid of mucous, it isn't a long-term cure for your sinus pain. However, it will provide temporary relief.

An Old Friend

My grandmother kept a jar of Vicks vapor rub next to her bed. If her sinuses got stuffed up or if she had a headache, she'd dab a little under her nose and at her temples. Almost instantly, she'd feel the congestion clear a little and she could breathe easier.

RATTLE AND HUM: SNORING

Whether you're the snorer or the snoree, snoring can wreak havoc on a good night's sleep. Although in most cases the sleep partner gets the brunt of the abuse, snoring can indicate a potentially harmful condition known as sleep apnea—a condition which literally deprives the brain of oxygen for a short time. In other words, the snorer stops breathing multiple times during the night. This deprives the person of the necessary deep level of sleep, so even though they are sleeping, the body isn't getting the rest it needs. If you have a chronic snoring problem (don't worry, your sleep partner will tell you), you may want to consult your physician.

Using a humidifier can end snoring caused by dry air.

Changing Positions

If you or your spouse only has an occasional snoring problem, you might have success if the snorer doesn't sleep on his or her back. Simply having the snorer turn on his side or stomach should let both of you sleep more soundly. You might try placing a pillow under the snorer's back so it is more difficult for him to roll over in his sleep.

Sometimes, a little levity can be the cure. Raising the head of your bed can help the snorer breath easier, thereby cutting back on the snoring. Try putting bricks or wood blocks under the legs of the bed. Simply placing an extra pillow under the snorer's head may only aggravate the problem.

Lighten Up

Probably the best cure for snoring is one that can benefit everyone: losing weight. Carrying excess weight puts pressure on the diaphragm, and adds fat to the neck and throat. Eating healthy and getting regular exercise is the best way to achieve overall health. So, losing weight won't just help you sleep better, it will help you look better and feel better, too.

A BARK AS BAD AS ITS BITE: WHOOPING COUGH

This disease responds well to the consumption of a half cup of black currents per day. Black currents are the best source of Gamma Linolenic Acid (GLA). The medical reasons are not clear why this seems to reduce the symptoms and assist the body in the healing process, but it was the way grandma handled the problem long before medical science had its medications.

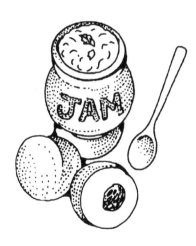

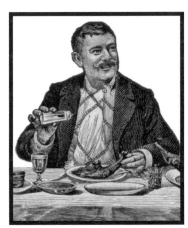

Chapter 11

HEART-Y HEALTH HINTS

ISN'T IT IRON-IC?: ANEMIA

Anemia is characterized by red blood cells (which are low in iron content) that are unable to carry sufficient oxygen to the body's tissues. Symptoms include weakness, loss of appetite, headaches, dizziness and depression.

Consume two tablespoons of blackstrap molasses daily to provide the iron needed for strong, healthy blood cells. Iron may also be found in a number of foods such as dark green leafy vegetables, raisins, prunes, beef and liver. Grandma's cupboard was never without a large jar of blackstrap molasses which she used to give to all the women just before and during their monthly cycle.

YOU GOTTA HAVE HEART: ARTERY HEALTH TEST

To test for good lower extremity circulation, see if you can feel the pulse directly behind the knee, at the top of the foot, or along the side of the ankle. Cayenne pepper improves blood flow and circulation.

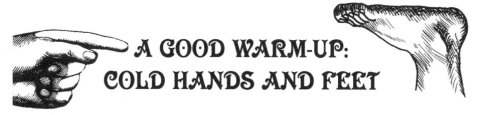

A GOOD WARM-UP: COLD HANDS AND FEET

Poor circulation to the extremities is a problem for many people.

Cold Hands, Warm Heart

If you've got cold hands and feet, you'll really warm up to this remedy. Grandma always said that a little cayenne pepper would do the trick. Cayenne tends to increase peripheral circulation and thus warm the extremities. Take one to two cayenne capsules.

Nutrient Know-How

Increasing your daily intake of Vitamin E can help a condition called intermittent claudation, which involves the narrowing of arteries in the legs. This condition may contribute to cold feet. To get Vitamin E into your diet, eat more vegetable oils, nuts, leafy green vegetables, and whole-grain cereals. You can also take a supplement, up to 400 IU daily. However, it's always a good idea to consult a doctor before starting any vitamin or mineral supplement.

• Heart-Y Health Hints •

Taking in more Niacin, one of the B vitamins, can increase blood supply to some parts of the body, causing the extremities to feel warmer. However, it generally takes a high dose to achieve this effect. Consult a doctor for a dosage that's right for you.

Tip-Toe Treatment

Increase circulation to your feet by doing stretches. Stand up on your toes for a couple of minutes and them come back down on your heels. Up and down, up and down, up and down, until you feel your feet tingling and the warmth coming back into them.

The Hot And Cold Solutions

To warm up your feet while you sleep, try the cold water cure. Fill your bath tub with a little cold water and walk back and forth for

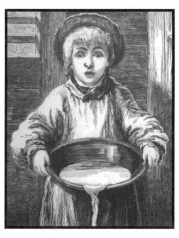

several minutes. Dry off your feet by rubbing them vigorously with a towel. You should be able to sleep through the night without feeling like you have icicles attached to your ankles.

Some people object to putting their chilled feet into cold water, even if it will make them feel better later. If that's true of you, soak your feet in hot water instead, with a cup of salt added to it. Bathe your feet for at least fifteen min-utes. Afterwards, dry your feet and mas-

sage with salt, for three to five minutes each, to improve circulation and remove dead skin cells. Rinse and dry feet again.

A Tingling Sensation

Put cayenne pepper into your socks to warm up cold feet. Just don't be surprised when your socks and skin turn red!

Apply this ginger-mustard paste to the bottoms of your feet to warm them up at night. Grate about an ounce of fresh ginger root. Put into a cheesecloth and squeeze out the juice. Mix it with two teaspoons of mustard powder. Leave it on your feet for fifteen minutes, using plastic bags to keep it from getting on the floor, the furniture, and everywhere else. Repeat this treatment for seven days in a row to relieve cold feet.

THE DROP ON "DROPSY": EDEMA

Grandmother called the buildup of fluids in the tissues "dropsy" because the problem normally occurs in the lower extremities, especially the ankles, although it may happen in any part of the body. It is caused by poor functioning of the kidneys, heart or liver. It may cause muscle pain and discomfort. Some fluid retention may be caused by allergic reactions.

Swell Herbs

To help reduce the swelling caused by fluid retention, Grandma used herbs, including alfalfa, dandelion root, garlic, kelp, marshmallow and parsley. A high fiber diet also helps.

Aloe vera gel or ointment has been used effectively to reduce facial swelling and cure cold sores. The aloe should be placed on a dressing and remain on the affected area for two to three hours.

ICICLE EXTREMITIES: FROSTBITE

Sage tea helps improve circulation, warming up the body. Brew the tea by adding a teaspoon of sage to a cup of boiling water, steep, and drink.

Chilly Scenes Of Winter

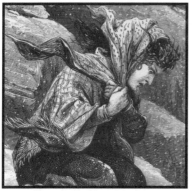

Grandma lived in Canada for a good part of her early life. Every winter, this preparation was always on the shelf and ready to use. In two cups of white wine, add one tablespoon white horseradish and one tablespoon fresh ginger root. Place two to three tablespoons of whole black peppercorns in the white wine solution. Strain well and place in a well-sealed jar in a cool, dark location until needed. Apply with a gentle touch using a very fine paint brush. The stinging pain associated with frostbite should be relieved almost instantly.

For mild frostbite, pour witch hazel over the affected area or apply olive oil with a cotton ball. Boil a pot of potatoes, mash, and add salt. Apply to the frostbitten area. You can also use the warm water in which you cooked the potatoes.

ALL PUMPED UP: HIGH BLOOD PRESSURE

Although not all causes of high blood pressure are known, some factors are obstruction of the arteries, increased fluid retention, kidney problems or stress.

The Daily Dose

Two tablespoons of flaxseed oil taken daily may lower high blood pressure.

• Heart-Y Health Hints •

Garlic has been used to lower blood pressure with excellent results. Roast three to four cloves of garlic daily and consume with food. Raw garlic will work just as well but has a potent taste that many people cannot tolerate.

The Japanese have long appreciated nutrient-rich kelp and have used it widely in their cooking and medicine. To the American palate, it's rather bad tasting. You can try eating kelp, or you can take powdered kelp or kelp pills. If you take a kelp supplement, be sure to follow the instructions on the package. Kelp is reputed to bring down high blood pressure.

Herbal Elixirs

A number of herbs have been used to successfully lower and regulate high blood pressure, including chamomile, hawthorn berries, hyssop and parsley. Take in the form of tea. Cayenne capsules are helpful, or drink two to three cups of summa herb tea daily.

Cayenne pepper is a powerful remedy for many ailments. Some research suggests that cayenne can also help lower blood pressure.

Watermelon seed has been quite successful in treating high blood pressure. If you want to make your own tea, take a couple teaspoons of the seed, crush them, and steep for an hour in a cup of boiling water. Strain the tea and drink a cup before each meal. You can also buy watermelon seed tea at most health food stores.

Another tea that can lower your blood pressure is raspberry leaf. Use an ounce of raspberry leaves to two cups of boiling water, allowing the tea to steep for twenty minutes. Take a cup of the brew every day.

Beneficial Bouquets

You know from personal experience that certain scents are relaxing and soothing. They may also be lifesaving. Some research suggests that the scent of the ocean, lavender and spicy apples may help lower blood pressure.

A Change Of Lifestyle

Cutting out salt can help lower blood pressure, especially in people who are sensitive to it. Most pre-packaged foods have tons of salt lurking in them, so be sure to read labels. You might want to make more meals from scratch, the way Grandma did, so you can control how much salt goes into your food.

You never can go wrong with exercise. Since being overweight is a contributing factor to high blood pressure, anything that brings weight down is helpful. Plus, studies show that people who exercise tend to have lower blood pressure than people who don't. Try taking a thirty-minute walk, four or five times a week.

If you like animals and have high blood pressure, get a pet. There's no scientific way to describe the effect petting a cat or dog or watching fish swim in an aquarium has on the human body and spirit, but it's a wonderful thing!

Drinking more water may help relieve hypertension. If you tend to drink other beverages when thirsty, try switching to water.

My grandmother's morning walk wasn't simply a matter of exercise. It was her meditation time, although she never called it that. Take some quiet time for yourself and relax, breathing deeply and slowly. This will temporarily lower your blood pressure. It's unclear whether meditation has any long-term benefits, but it certainly can't hurt.

Keeping The Doctor Away

An apple, or two, really can keep you out of the doctor's office, if you have high blood pressure, that is. Try to eat two apples every day to lower blood pressure. The pectin, a natural fiber found in apples, appears to provide the beneficial effect.

My grandmother served fish several times a week. She was convinced it's good for whatever ails you. Many people believe that eating more fish can help bring down high blood pressure. Most types of fish are low in fat, which is good for anyone concerned about blood pressure or heart problems.

Potassium Power

Too little potassium in the diet can cause high blood pressure. Try eating dried apricots, lima beans, pinto beans, potatoes with their skins on, and bananas. You can also take supplements, but you should check with your doctor to determine the dosage.

Cucumbers are rich in potassium, as well as other minerals. They also have a calming effect, which helps bring down blood pressure. Try to eat at least one cucumber everyday. You can also take them in the form of juice if you own a juicer. Drink a half cup of cucumber juice daily.

For a high-potassium tea that should help lower blood pressure, boil unpeeled potatoes for fifteen minutes. Drink two cups of the cooled liquid every day.

• *Heart-Y Health Hints* •

Cajun Cure

Under the category of leap-of-faith cures comes this down-home Louisiana remedy for lowering blood pressure. Place pieces of Spanish moss, a plant found in abundance in bayou territory, in your shoes and walk around in them. Of course, there's no scientific reason to believe this will work, but you can be sure there will be no negative side-effects.

CLOGGING UP THE WORKS: HIGH CHOLESTEROL

This is a fatty substance found in animal products that causes buildup in arteries. It is one of the major causes of stroke and heart disease. The majority of cholesterol is produced by the liver and is essential to the building of cell membranes and sex hormones.

The Daily Allowance

Taking 500 IU of Vitamin E a day can boost the level of good cholesterol, helping to bring the bad cholesterol under control. It has positive effects on other cardiovascular conditions as well. Check with your doctor before trying this remedy and ask about the optimal dosage for you.

Niacin will definitely reduce cholesterol levels, however you should check with a doctor before taking supplements since excess amounts of this B-vitamin can be harmful.

The amount of chromium in the system appears to effect the body's cholesterol level. People who do not get enough chromium may be more susceptible to high cholesterol. You can take brewer's yeast or eat sunflower seeds, like my Grandma, to get more chromium in your diet. You can also take a supplement. Your doctor can recommend the appropriate dosage.

Nature's Cholesterol Cutters

A number of herbs may be used to lower cholesterol levels, including cayenne in capsule form and teas made from goldenseal and hawthorn berries.

Taking raw, chopped garlic has positive effects on high cholesterol. Raw is definitely better than cooked. Chop it very fine, and hide it in your food or wash it down with plenty of water. Garlic can help reduce the level of fat in the blood.

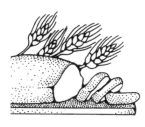

Fiber Is Our Friend

Oat bran bread and muffins are an excellent source of the type of fiber that binds cholesterol and carries the excess out of the body.

Pectin, a natural fiber found in certain fruits, appears to aid in lowering cholesterol. Eat more grapefruit and apples. To actually get the pectin, leave the peel on the apple and eat the white stuff on the flesh of the grapefruit.

The Virtue Of Vegetables

Certain vegetables help reduce bad cholesterol. If you're trying to bring your cholesterol level down, eat more brussel sprouts, broccoli, rutabagas, eggplants, and turnips.

Carrots appear to be especially effective in reducing cholesterol. Try to eat two to three raw carrots a day.

Drink lots of fresh vegetable and fruit juice to lower cholesterol. It's low in fat, and the natural fiber pectin helps prevent cholesterol from being absorbed into the blood.

Bet On Beans

Beans taste good, they're an important part of a balanced diet, and they do a lot to lower cholesterol. You can eat any variety you like in any form that makes you happy. Try some lentil soup for lunch, roasted corn and black bean salsa with low-fat chips for your next snack, or lima beans as a side dish with your favorite dinner. Make beans a part of your regular diet for a low-cholesterol life.

Eating soybeans and its products can help bring down your cholesterol level. If you'd just rather not, you can take lecithin, a soybean derivative, instead. It comes in many forms—capsules, liquid, tablets. You can find lecithin at your local pharmacy or health food store.

Don't Be A Couch Potato

If you have high cholesterol, try getting thirty minutes of aerobic exercise, at least three or four times a week. This level of activity increases good cholesterol that clears out arteries and reduces the bad stuff.

A TANGLED WEB: VARICOSE VEINS

Varicose veins are caused by the breakdown of valves located at intervals inside the veins which allow blood to flow back to the heart. This condition may be hereditary or may be caused by sitting for prolonged periods without leg movement. Swelling may occur which causes the valves to stop working and the veins to become stretched from pressure.

Preventive Measures

To keep from getting, or aggravating, varicose veins, don't cross your legs or wear socks or stockings that can constrict blood flow at a certain point on your legs.

Wearing support hose will prevent varicose veins from becoming worse and will ease pain. Make sure that they are tightest around the ankle and get gradually looser as they go up the leg. You'll feel like your legs are getting a massage all day long.

Internal Medicine

Increase foods in your diet that are high in vitamin K and E such as blackstrap molasses and dark green leafy vegetables. Check with your doctor for the appropriate dosage.

Taking one aspirin a day will reduce or even eliminate varicose veins for some people.

Some have found relief from vinegar. Mix two tablespoons apple cider vinegar with three tablespoon of water and one pint warm water. Take two ounces of the mixture every day. If you're beginning to develop varicose veins, this remedy may help prevent them.

Herbal Essentials

An ancient cure for varicose veins was to use the herb bayberry bark. A solution is made by making some strong bayberry tea and dipping a type of very absorbent terry cloth towel into the mixture then applying the towel over the area that is affected. The towel with the solution should be as hot as the person will tolerate and then covered with another cloth to help retain the heat for a longer period of time. A heating pad may even be placed over the dry towel.

191

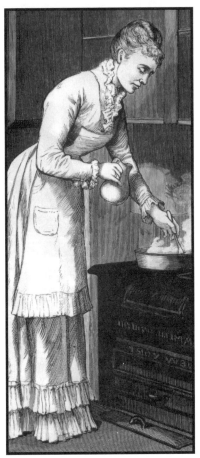

The herb calendula has also had remarkable effects on varicose veins. The herb must be prepared in the following manner and placed on a cloth which is then wrapped around the leg and allowed to remain for two to three hours at a time. This should be done twice a day for about four weeks. The ointment can be prepared by using eight ounces of fresh calendura flowers, leaves and stems. Place two to three cups of lard in a skillet, heat and add the diced calendura. Remove the skillet from the heat and allow to stand for twelve hours. Warm the mixture up and strain through a filter and place the mixture in a jar until needed.

Massage your legs with tincture of arnica, an herbal preparation you can buy at most health food stores. It helps reduce pain and swelling. Rubbing your legs will help move blood out of your legs and back up to the heart, preventing blood vessels from ballooning and breaking.

Speed Up, Slow Down

Exercise is always recommended, but regular exercise can keep varicose veins from getting worse—or showing up at all. Try exercises that don't put a lot of stress on your legs, such as swimming, walking or bicycling.

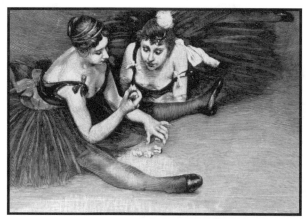

If you have varicose veins, it's important to get off your feet regularly. Try lying down or sitting with your legs extended in front of you for fifteen minutes out of every hour. This treats the primary culprit of varicose veins: gravity.

Shrink Wrap It

Apple cider vinegar can help to shrink varicose veins. Make a bandage from cheesecloth and soak it in apple cider vinegar. Wrap the cheesecloth around the area. Lie on your back, raise your legs and relax for half an hour. When you're done, drink two teaspoons of apple cider vinegar in a cup of warm water. Do this twice a day— once in the morning and once at night. You may see a noticeable difference in a few weeks.

You can reduce the swelling of varicose veins by making a bandage out of cheesecloth, soaking it in witch hazel and wrapping it around the affected area. It will work even better if you lie down and raise your legs for several minutes.

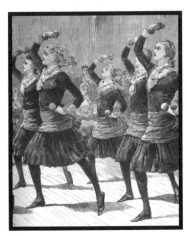

Chapter 12

WHEN YOUR INNARDS
AIL YOU...

FIXING THE FURNACE:
BODY TEMPERATURE

The body's temperature is controlled by the hypothalamus gland. It has warmth detector cells that monitor hot and cold levels. One very hot summer day, I saw a woman eating chili peppers and asked her why. I thought it would increase body heat due to the chemical capsaicin it contains. To my surprise, the woman explained that capsicin controls the hypothalamus mechanism and will actually keep the body cooler on a hot day. She also mentioned that this method of body cooling is used in many countries around the world, especially African nations and other equatorial regions.

SUGAR RUSH: DIABETES

This disease is characterized by the inability of the body to breakdown sugars for use by the body's cells. When this mechanism breaks down, an abnormal amount of sugar or glucose ends up in the bloodstream and causes problems with almost all systems in the body. Sugar levels need to be regulated so that they remain relatively constant. Many people who suffer from diabetes can be helped with a number of herbs and a well balanced-diet.

Don't Overlook A Deficiency

Scientific research has shown that insufficient amounts of chromium, a trace mineral that the body needs, contributes to the onset of diabetes in adults. The mineral appears to increase insulin efficiency. Many people seem to suffer from chromium deficiency. To avoid it, eat foods high in chromium, including broccoli, other vegetables, fruits, whole grains, and brewer's yeast. You can also take a supplement of fifty milligrams daily.

Deficiency of the vitamin B6 may contribute to diabetes. Since an excess of this vitamin can cause serious problems, check with your doctor if this treatment is appropriate for you and what the proper dose should be.

Dietary "Dos"

In addition to following a careful diet, make a salad out of fresh garlic, parsley, and watercress to eat every day. This combination may help normalize your blood sugar level.

Add Jerusalem artichokes to your diet to help control diabetes. It's possible that this vegetable helps the body produce insulin. Jerusalem artichokes taste sweet, like yams, and making them a regular part of your diet can help satisfy sugar cravings. This vegetable is also quite nutritious, containing lots of vitamins and minerals, and is low in fat and calories.

Legumes should be an integral part of any diabetic's nutrition plan. All varieties of bean, from black beans to lima, are high in fiber and low in fat. They also help reduce bad cholesterol and blood sugar levels.

Hoofing It

Reducing weight is a key measure in treating diabetes. Of course, exercise is a significant part of any weight loss program. Start gently and gradually increase strenuousness as your fitness level improves. Walking is a great low-impact activity. Thirty minutes of exercise every other day, in combination with the proper diet, can help you lose weight, and you'll feel great!

From The Herbal Pharmacy

One of the most effective herbs in the regulation of blood sugar levels is Korean ginseng. The combination of a balanced complex carbohydrate diet and two Korean ginseng capsules a day or ginseng tea has done wonders for many people who are not insulin dependent.

There are several herbal teas that can help reduce blood sugar levels and stabilize a diabetic condition. Take two to four cups of yarrow tea daily. You can intersperse doses of yarrow tea with dandelion tea or blueberry leaf tea. You can find dried dandelion leaves or root, as well as blueberry leaves, at your local health food store. It is also beneficial to eat fresh dandelion greens. They make a zingy, tasty addition to a salad.

Sage Advice

Sage tea has traditionally been recommended for a variety of ailments. It helps those with diabetes feel better and may help reduce blood sugar level. Brew one dose with one tablespoon sage leaves and one cup boiling water. Take up to three cups a day.

A STONE'S THROW: GALLBLADDER PROBLEMS

The gall bladder is a reservoir for bile salts used by the body to dissolve fats. Stones may develop causing severe pain. Symptoms usually occur after a person has eaten a high-fat meal.

Cleanse the gallbladder using oil of peppermint capsules. Other effective herbs include catnip, dandelion, fennel, parsley and wild yam. Barberry root bark prepared as a tea is also helpful.

Olive oil seems to be the remedy of choice for helping your body get rid of gallstones. Warm half a cup of virgin olive oil and drink it slowly while lying on the floor. Or make yourself an olive oil cocktail for breakfast, by adding two tablespoon of pure virgin olive oil to half a cup grapefruit juice.

How Does It Feel?: Like A Rolling Stone

A cure for gallstones has been handed down in my family for many years. Consume apple cider vinegar in half cup portions, four to five times a day for four days. Please note: This is the only liquid you are allowed. During the third and fourth days, you need to drink three of the drinks with only a quarter cup of vinegar and a quarter cup of olive oil added. By the fifth day you should pass the stones.

The "Gall" Of Black Radish

In Grandma's garden, you'd find a row of black radishes. She grew them specifically to help Grandpa's gallbladder troubles. When it started acting up on him, she'd grate some of the radishes and use a piece of cloth to squeeze out the juice. She'd give Grandpa a dose before each meal, no more than two tablespoons at a time. Grandpa would feel better within a couple of weeks and go back to his usual routine without any symptoms.

The Energizer

Gall bladder problems can really sap your energy. If you can't seem to get started, try this zingy pick-me-up. First thing in the morning, drink half a glass of warm water with the juice of one lemon squeezed into it. After a week, you should feel more like your old self.

ALL REVVED UP: HYPERTHYROIDISM

This disorder of the thyroid gland, where too much hormone is produced, results in an increase in metabolism. The symptoms include nervousness, irritability, insomnia, and fatigue.

Reduce consumption of dairy products and increase intake of soybeans, cabbage, spinach, brussel sprouts, kale and mustard greens.

ENERGY CRISIS: HYPOGLYCEMIA

Low blood sugar is caused by oversecretion of insulin by the pancreas. Symptoms include dizziness, fatigue, irritability, headaches, anxiety and depression. Weakness in the lower extremities is also common.

A diet high in complex carbohydrates, with snacks of high-protein food between meals, helps to regulate blood sugar levels.

FEELING SLUGGISH: HYPOTHYROIDISM

This condition occurs when the thyroid gland is unable to produce sufficient quantities of the necessary hormone. Symptoms are fatigue, muscle weakness, obesity, and possibly an orange discoloration of the skin.

Teas made from goldenseal, bayberry, and black cohosh aid this condition. These herbs mimic the missing hormone and fool the body into thinking sufficient levels are present.

SECURITY ALERT: THE IMMUNE SYSTEM

An effective immune system enhancer is a soup made from the herb astragulus, along with shiitake and maitake mushrooms. Use several slices of astragulus and a handful of dried mushrooms. Add them to your

favorite homemade soup recipe. The soup should simmer for approximately one hour. The ingredients can be found in most Asian food
stores, markets or health food shops.

Raw garlic appears to have significant immune enhancing properties. However, the active ingredient "allicin" may be destroyed if
cooked. Try pickled garlic which is less pungent then the raw bulb.

THE YELLOW SCARE: JAUNDICE

Jaundice is a buildup of bilirubin, a yellow-brown substance in the
blood that is not removed through the normal cleansing process per-
formed by the liver. The "back-up" in the blood causes the skin to
have a yellow-orange color. Urine becomes darker and the whites of
the eyes may also have a yellow tint. Jaundice is usually related to
liver disease.

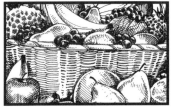

Try changing your diet so that you are
eating seventy percent raw fruits and vegetables. Follow this plan for three weeks.

To remedy this condition, drink either
one cup lemon juice and water three times a day, or drink beet juice
made with the tops juiced as well, taking one cup three times a day
for five days.

FILTER FAILURES: KIDNEY PROBLEMS

One of the more common kidney/bladder problems relates to the
breakdown of the filtration system. Waste products spill over into
the blood and are not excreted efficiently. Infections are common and
may result in fever.

A lack of magnesium can lead to a chronic problem with kidney stones. A recommended daily dosage is 600 milligrams of magnesium taken with 25 milligrams of vitamin B6. You should consult your doctor for the dosage that is optimal for you.

Flooding Your System

Grandma believed that drinking plenty of water was the foundation of good health. If you have problems with kidney stones, it's great advice. Getting plenty of water keeps the fluids passing through the kidneys safely diluted, so stones are less likely to form. How much water you need each day depends on your climate and level of exertion, since sweating releases fluids from the body.

Consume one quart of marshmallow root tea daily. Cranberry tea and watermelon seed are also effective.

Unsweetened cranberry juice increases the acidity of the urine, slowing the growth of bacteria. Drink at least three eight ounce glasses a day.

Shrinking A Stone

Depending on the kind of kidney stone you have, baking soda may be an effective remedy. For uric acid and cystine stones, take a teaspoon of baking soda in eight ounces of water, four times a day, for a week or so. Check with your doctor to see if this is a good treatment for you. Remember that baking soda is high in sodium, and you should steer clear of it if you're watching your salt intake.

A Clean Sweep

An old remedy for kidney and bladder problems is to consume five cloves of garlic a day. Garlic has long been known as a cleansing herb.

Eat parsnips. They are a great detoxifier and can help clean your kidneys.

Infection Fighter

If you have an infection, flaxseed can help you fight it. Make flaxseed tea by steeping one tablespoon of flaxseed in one pint of boiling water. Steep for seven minutes and strain.

GOOD HOUSEKEEPING: LIVER CLEANSING

The liver can be cleansed using a combination of black radish and dandelion.

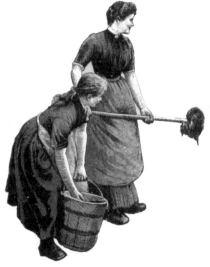

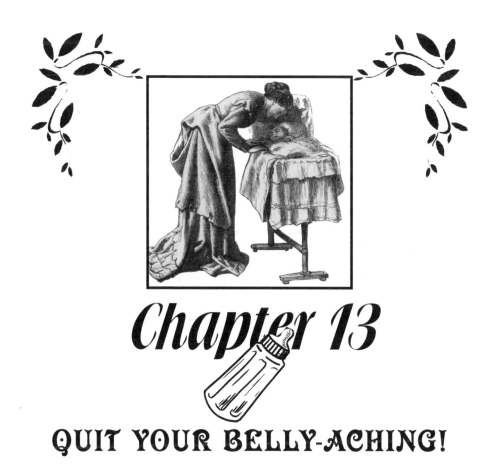

Chapter 13

QUIT YOUR BELLY-ACHING!

LETTING THE AIR OUT: COLIC

Colic is probably caused by intestinal gas. Symptoms include crying, clenched fists, bulging abdominal area and whining.

There are many benefits to breast feeding your baby. Breast milk contains the nutrients a baby needs, boosts the child's immunity, and lets you snuggle and bond with your baby. However, if you eat dairy products, your breast milk may cause colic in your child. Experiment with your diet, eliminating dairy and getting the calcium you need

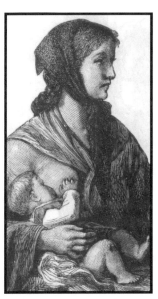

from other sources, such as whole grains and green leafy vegetables. This remedy works in about half the cases of colic.

Grandma's Rock-A-Bye Baby Method

When babysitting for colicky infants, Grandma used to place one to two ounces of ginger ale into their bottles. She said this would soothe the discomfort almost all of the time. The carbonation helps the release of gas. Try and get the baby to burp on your shoulder. This will also solve the problem. Grandma's favorite remedy: Rock the baby in a rocking chair.

Baby's Belly Brews

Brew a tea of one teaspoon fennel seed and a quarter teaspoon sugar. Cool, strain, and pour into your child's bottle. It will calm the baby and help get rid of gas.

Add one ounce fresh peppermint leaves to a pint of boiling water and steep. The peppermint tea should be lukewarm when given to the child. A quarter cup will usually ease the symptoms and help the child sleep. You can also try letting your child suck on a peppermint stick. Not all children can tolerate peppermint's pungent taste. If your baby has trouble with it, try another remedy.

Make a tea from caraway seeds to soothe a colicky baby. Steep a tablespoon of caraway seeds in a cup of boiling water for ten minutes. Cool and strain out the seeds. A couple of teaspoons should be enough to ease gas pains and soothe the infant. You can give it to the baby in a bottle.

The Tried And True

Put corn syrup on your child's pacifier to help ease colic, or add a quarter teaspoon brown sugar to an eight ounce bottle of milk. It should help the baby expel gas. Of course, you don't want to overdo the sugar. That won't be good for the baby's teeth.

My grandmother found that simple cures were often quite effective. Warmth will help soothe a colicky baby. Try filling a hot water bottle with warm, not hot, water and place on the child's stomach. Or you can just hold your baby close and soothe the child with the warmth of your body and your loving touch.

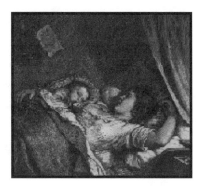

White Noise Works

Grandma had a way with children. Neighbors with colicky babies would bring them over to get her help. She would tell them to take the baby for a long buggy ride, and that would do the trick every time. The child would stop crying and usually fall asleep. The repetitive motion and noise, not the horse, were the important parts. Try wrapping your baby in a blanket and put the child in a laundry basket. Place the basket next to your clothes dryer and turn it on for twenty minutes. Vacuuming in the child's presence may also help your baby relax. The vibration can help the baby's intestine do its work, relieving gas and easing the colic.

FRIDGE FRIGHT: FOOD POISONING

Here's an antidote for food poisoning from bad shellfish. Bring two pints of water to a rapid boil, add two teaspoons cherry bark, one tablespoon fresh, grated ginger root and one finely diced onion. Allow the mixture to simmer ten minutes, remove from heat and allow to steep for thirty minutes. Drink two cups while it is still warm.

A RAGING INFERNO: HEARTBURN

This burning sensation in the abdomen is related to the excess release of hydrochloric acid, causing irritation to the stomach lining and the esophagus. Certain foods and liquids can cause this reaction, including coffee (more than two cups a day), alcohol, carbonated beverages, citrus fruits, tomato products and certain spices.

Tranquil Tummy Teas

A tea made from ginger soothes the stomach and controls the excess release of acid.

Slippery elm bark has been used for many years to ease an acid stomach and relieve heartburn discomfort. Look for this herb at your local health food store. You can use the bark itself or a powder made from it, one teaspoon of either in a cup of boiling water. Sip the tea, and you should feel better shortly.

Undoing A Sugar Overdose

You know how kids are. They love sweet stuff, and sometimes they don't know when to quit. That's exactly the way I was as a child, especially at Grandma's house where there were so many delicious treats waiting for me in her kitchen. Whenever I ate too many of her goodies, Grandma would shake her head and say, "Poor thing. You've got a sore tummy, don't you?" Then she'd whip up her favorite remedy to settle a stomach sick from eating too many sugary sweets. She'd mix a cup of warm water, the juice of half a lemon, and a teaspoon of salt. She'd put her arm around me and tell me to drink it down slowly. It wasn't very long before I was feeling much better and looking for my next cookie.

Chew On This

Sometimes you can chew your way to heartburn relief. Take a mouthful of dry oats and chew until it's soft enough to swallow. Your favorite chewing gum can also reduce stomach acid and prevent heartburn.

Eating six unblanched almonds, chewing them very slowly and thoroughly, can help reduce acid in the stomach and soothe the discomfort.

You can also eat raw carrots to counteract heartburn. Peel them and chew each bite slowly and thoroughly.

Make-It-Better Beverages

Place one raw potato, that has been thoroughly washed with the skin still on, in a juicer. Dilute the juice evenly with water and drink three times a day. The potato juice must be made fresh.

Grandma preferred leaf lettuce to iceberg, but she always grew some iceberg lettuce to use in her heartburn remedy. Puree a few lettuce leaves and three quarters cup cold water in your blender. Sip the green liquid and prepare for relief.

One tablespoon raw apple cider vinegar mixed with cold water and sipped slowly during a meal is an effective treatment. Do not consume any other liquid with your meal.

This remedy sounds like it would do more to upset your stomach than settle it, but many people swear by it. Combine an egg white with two tablespoons of olive oil and drink all of the mixture.

Simple But Effective

Activated charcoal is highly absorbent. Take a capsule of it to absorb the excess stomach acid that causes heartburn.

Drink a glass of water with a teaspoon of baking soda dissolved in it. It will help neutralize acid in the stomach. Don't use too much baking soda or use this remedy after an especially large meal, since it's full of salt and can create too much pressure in the stomach.

Feel The Burn? Reach For Peppermint!

Grandpa loved to eat. Grandma was a wonderful cook, so they had a very happy marriage. Unfortunately, Grandpa could sometimes overdo it at the dinner table and end up with heartburn. Grandma would make him walk around the house to keep the blood moving so he could digest all that food, while she made him a nice, warm cup of tea from peppermint leaves she had grown in her garden. The peppermint soothed Grandpa's stomach, and pretty soon, he'd be ready for dessert.

SPELLING RELIEF: INDIGESTION

This condition is usually a stomach disorder, but may also relate to the small or large intestine. Symptoms include bloating, flatulence, abdominal pain, belching, a burning sensation or nausea. The problem may occur from consuming liquids with meals. This neutralizes enzymes that are needed to break down foods.

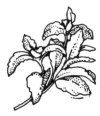 These herbs are useful in alleviating symptoms: mint, papaya, peppermint, chamomile and fennel. For inflammation of the colon, an enema using the herb slippery elm should provide fast relief.

Before The Burn

You may know that there are certain foods that always seem to irritate your stomach. Foods that are hard to digest, or foods that produce gas often cause stomach problems, or aggravate existing conditions. If you just can't resist, try taking an activated charcoal capsule along with the culprit food. Another option is to take one tablespoonful of olive oil before you eat. You may find that you can then enjoy hot or irritating foods without the discomfort.

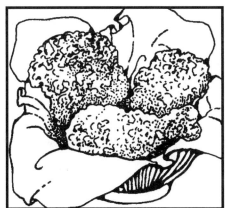

If you like vegetables, but they don't like you, there's no need to despair. Just sprinkle fresh lemon juice on vegetables more than three hours before you plan to eat them. This marinade makes the veggies easier to digest. It also adds a nice flavor.

If you're going to serve a hard-to-digest meal, this side dish does double duty. Steam some zucchini and sprinkle with raw, grated almonds. It's tasty and will aid in digestion.

A Japanese radish called daikon is a wonderful digestive aid. It's crisp, refreshing and very effective, especially when eating oily or fried foods. You can add raw daikon to salads. Grate one or two tablespoons, or eat a few slices with your meal.

Here's a hot tip for indigestion sufferers: cayenne pepper. Sprinkle some (not too much) on all kinds of food and it will help in digestion.

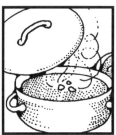

Grandma's Brown Rice And Fresh Barley Belly Soup

A soup made from brown rice and fresh barley should help alleviate bloating and flatulence. Boil five parts water to one part of the grain mixture for ten to twelve minutes and then allow to simmer for forty-five minutes before straining. Allow to cool before consuming.

Natural Acid Neutralizers

Papaya is another natural cure for stomach pain. This tropical fruit has long been recognized for its qualities as a digestive aid. After eating, take papaya—you can drink papaya juice, eat the fresh fruit or take papaya pills. Most health food stores will carry a number of brands of papaya products to choose from. Check them out and see which works best for you.

For acid ingestion, you may find kelp tablets to be a welcome relief. Kelp is a form of seaweed which forms a gel that soothes upset stomachs by binding up stomach acid. A caution to those who must watch their salt intake: this is not the cure for you. Kelp (and other seaweed) is very high in sodium.

How about a spicy solution to your stomach ache? Try chewing cardamom seeds. This fragrant spice has long been recognized as a digestive aid. Chewing cardamom seeds can relieve nausea, discomfort and help to relieve gas buildup. Plus, it has a pleasant flavor. Other fragrant spices can be helpful too. Try anise seeds and caraway seeds. They'll help your stomach, and like the cardamom seeds, they can sweeten your breath.

If you suffer from acid indigestion, try chewing a teaspoon of dry rolled oats. Make sure you chew the oats thoroughly before you swallow. They will help to soothe you and neutralize the acid in your stomach.

Grandma's Grapefruit Granules

Grandma's herb garden and her abundance of home remedies gained her some notoriety with her friends and neighbors. This is one that a lot of her friends took on as their own. I'm sure they passed this remedy on to their family, so there are probably an awful lot of medicine cabinets around the country that contain a jar of Grandma's grapefruit granule. It's a remedy you can prepare well in advance for when an upset stomach strikes. Grate a grapefruit peel, and let the shavings dry on a paper towel. Once they are completely dry, place them in a jar with a tight lid and place the jar in your medicine cabinet. The dried peel keeps very well. So, the next time your stomach is upset, reach for the jar and chew a teaspoon of the peel. Make sure you chew very well, and get the granules saturated with saliva. You'll thank Grandma, just like her friends and neighbors used to.

Tea-rrific Tummy Ache Tamers

To settle your stomach, boil one teaspoon of alfalfa seed in one cup of water. Let the seeds steep for approximately five minutes. Strain and drink the tea a half an hour after your meal.

If you have stomach discomfort from overeating, drinking fenugreek tea can make you feel better in no time. Crush one teaspoon of the seeds in a cup of boiling water and steep for approximately five minutes. Strain the crushed fenugreek seeds and sip.

Sipping a cup of sage tea can help get rid of the bad breath and the white coating on the tongue that can come along with an upset stomach.

• Quit Your Belly-Aching! •

If you suffer from a nervous stomach, try this soothing tea. Take a half teaspoon of dried marjoram and a quarter teaspoon of dried oregano and steep for ten minutes in one cup of hot water. Strain the herbs and slowly sip the tea. You may repeat in two hours if the first cup doesn't do the trick.

Other teas that will help your upset stomach are chamomile and peppermint. Drink a cup at the first sign of discomfort and continue to sip as needed.

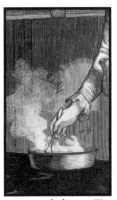

Cookin' Up A Cure

This is a home remedy that may be a little difficult to take, but it really seems to work. At the first sign of stomach discomfort, boil one sliced onion in one cup of milk. Drink this while it's still warm. It's difficult, but it's better than the stomach pain.

Another way to neutralize acid is to drink raw potato juice. To make the juice, grate a potato and squeeze (it's best to squeeze through cheesecloth if you have it). One tablespoon diluted in half a cup of warm water should make you feel better. Be sure to drink it slowly.

Sometimes overeating can bring on a sensation known as a "sour stomach". Or, you may feel that something you've eaten "doesn't agree with you." Here's a quick remedy that many people find helpful for settling their stomach. Add one teaspoon of apple cider vinegar to a glass of water. If the sour taste is too much for you, you may want to add some honey.

Speaking of honey, this natural nectar has been found to bring sweet relief to some stomach pain sufferers. A tablespoon or two of honey can do wonders to relieve stomach cramps. This is no new-fangled remedy—the appreciation of honey's curative qualities dates all the way back to ancient Egypt.

• Quit Your Belly-Aching! •

Tartar For The Tummy

When I was a child, Grandma would give me cream of tartar in water whenever I had a stomach ache. She always had it on hand for baking and it always made me feel better (after a good belch or two).

To settle our stomachs, she would also make us arrowroot paste—arrowroot is terrific for settling the stomach. Make the paste by combining one tablespoon of arrowroot with enough water to get the right consistency. Mix until smooth. Then, boil, cool and add one tablespoon of fresh lime juice.

Without Sugar Or Spice

For stomach ailments, many doctors recommend the BRAT diet. This works particularly well if you have the stomach flu. It's a bland diet that consists of foods that are easy to take on an upset stomach: Bananas, Rice, Applesauce and Toast. Easy to remember, easy to digest.

Shower Yourself With Relief

Sometimes just a hot shower is all you need to feel better. Let the hot shower water run on your stomach. You should feel better—and more relaxed within ten to fifteen minutes.

WHEN THE ROOM IS SPINNING: MOTION SICKNESS

This order is caused by conflicting signals sent to the brain through the vestibule apparatus in the ear and sensory nerves.

Take four to five charcoal tablets approximately one hour before a trip. Ginger capsules are just as good, but you need to take two to

213

three capsules one hour before the trip, then every three hours thereafter.

On The Road

Whatever the mode of transportation, sit near a window and look out, focusing on faraway objects. If that doesn't work, try sucking on a lemon.

Some people believe that the delicate skin on your inner wrist can send a signal to your brain to let up on the motion sickness. Grab the skin on your inner wrist (just an inch below your palm) and pull on it and pinch. Keep it up until you feel better—be sure to alternate wrists.

When you start feeling queasy, it's important to get fresh air. If you're traveling by car, train or bus, open a window and breath deeply. If you're on a boat, stay on deck. Open the overhead fan on a plane.

Motion Potions

If you get seasick, try taking marjoram tea. Drink a cup of tea before getting on board ship.

You can also try peppermint or chamomile tea. Both are excellent for soothing the stomach and relieving nausea.

Not quite so soothing a thought is this peppery drink. In a cup of warm water, mix an eighth teaspoon of cayenne pepper. Drink it all—you can hold your nose, if you like.

BELLY FLOPS: NAUSEA

If you're finding it difficult to eat, try peeling and eating half a cucumber. It will feel very soothing and refreshing and won't irritate your system.

Tummy Tonics

Fresh ginger or ginger capsules seem to reduce nausea and even eliminate it in many cases. In some countries, ginger powder is actually prescribed after surgery to alleviate the nausea from anesthesia.

Try placing a few drops of peppermint tincture under your tongue. The queasy feeling should go away in a few minutes. You can find a large variety of herbal tinctures at health food stores.

Peppermint tea is another herbal alternative to ease stomach discomfort. If you don't have the tea handy, try a peppermint candy.

Chamomile tea is a popular remedy for an upset stomach. There are many brands of chamomile tea that you can find in any grocery store or health food store. Chamomile tea is also very soothing and can help when you feel stress. It's great before bedtime, too. Note: if you are sensitive to ragweed, chrysanthemums or aster, you should avoid chamomile.

Yarrow tea can provide quick relief from nausea. Drink one cup when you start to get that queasy feeling. Cloves, cinnamon stick and ginger are all good for stopping nausea. Steep a couple of cloves in boiling water for five minutes, or try cinnamon stick, or one teaspoon of powdered ginger. Any one of these teas will help to ease your nausea.

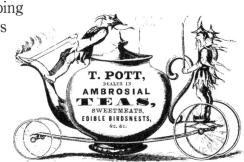

T. POTT,
DEALER IN
AMBROSIAL
TEAS,
SWEETMEATS,
EDIBLE BIRDSNESTS,
&c. &c.

From The Soda Fountain

Believe it or not, soda can help relieve nausea. Sipping ginger ale is a good preventive measure for nausea. You might also try Coca-Cola for an upset stomach. Cola syrup is also terrific for nausea. You can easily find this over-the-counter-item at your pharmacy. One teaspoon of this sweet syrup works very well.

Chewing on ice chips can also curb nausea.

Bumpy Ride Candy

Whenever we would travel long distances, Grandma always kept candies in her purse. Her favorite was barley sugar, and she always had a supply handy for long, bumpy rides. Any hard candy is a good deterrent for car sickness, but sugar always reminds me of Grandma. The best thing about this remedy is that if your kids get car sickness, you won't have to talk them into taking their medicine!

Managing Morning Sickness

Taking two or three capsules of powdered ginger root each morning can help you avoid morning sickness altogether.

Another morning sickness remedy is vitamin B-6. It is most effective for women who have severe morning sickness (vomiting several times a day). Check with your doctor before you start taking the vitamins because like many vitamins, taking too much B-6 can be harmful.

Nausea caused by morning sickness can often be allayed by eating crackers. Many women swear by saltines. Keep a box in the car, and even keep some in your purse. When that feeling comes over you, you'll be glad you have them handy.

If you suffer from morning sickness, you may get some relief from drinking one teaspoon of bicarbonate of soda in a half a glass of water. Or, try drinking carbonated mineral water.

A SORE SPOT: ULCERS

Ulcers may occur anywhere along the gastrointestinal tract, however, they are more common in the stomach when the stomach is unable to secrete sufficient quantities of mucous to protect the delicate lining from the hydrochloric acid.

Prevention is the key when it comes to ulcers. If you suffer from ulcer pain, avoiding the following foods could keep your suffering at bay: milk, fried foods, spicy foods, acidic foods and fatty foods. While these foods don't cause ulcers, avoiding them may keep you from getting a flare-up.

Although you should avoid spicy foods, cayenne pepper is a very helpful spice to use in ulcer healing. Drink an eighth teaspoon of cayenne pepper in a glass of water twice daily. If you can stand it, work your way up to a quarter teaspoon of the pepper.

A Dairy Don't

Never drink milk to soothe the stomach. The calcium in milk tends to stimulate the production of additional acid. The only milk that may be helpful is almond milk.

Soothing Stomach Savers

Ulcers respond well to a tea made from chamomile or bayberry. Cayenne capsules also tend to promote healing by increasing circulation.

• Quit Your Belly-Aching! •

Some people find that gingerroot can calm an ulcer flare-up. Licorice has been known to have the same effect. A variety known as DGL, deglycyrrhized licorice, is available in health food stores and can help protect the stomach's lining.

Drinking catnip tea before each meal can make a noticeable difference for many stomach ulcer sufferers. Either use a tea bag, or one teaspoon of catnip in a cup of boiling water. Let steep for five minutes, strain and drink.

Rejuvenate With Juice

Fresh cabbage juice will ease the problem but needs to be consumed immediately after juicing before oxidation has a chance to reduce its potency.

An extremely effective remedy is to take one tablespoon of aloe vera juice after each meal.

Whole Grain Goodness

Try this barley water remedy, but you might want to check with your doctor first. To six cups of water, add two ounces of pearled barley and boil down until only about half of the liquid remains in the pot. Strain the barley (it can be used for cooking) and drink. You may add honey and lemon to taste.

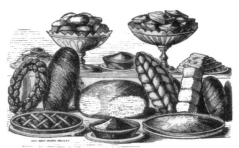

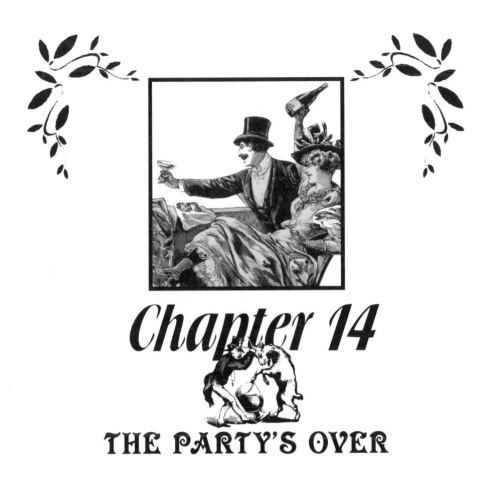

Chapter 14

THE PARTY'S OVER

ONE MORE ROUND:
ALCOHOL DEPENDENCY

A healthy, nourished body is the foundation of all wellness.
Beating alcoholism takes a change in lifestyle. It may be easier
if you eat more healthily, getting most of your daily intake of calories
from whole grains, vegetables, and fruits. Try to cut out all high-fat,
sugary, and processed foods that may contribute to your alcohol cravings.

Herbal Easers

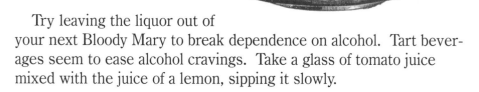

It will make the process of breaking someone's alcohol dependency easier if you can ease their cravings for alcohol. The herb angelica, either the roots or leaves, has properties that seem to lessen the desire for alcohol. A person who is trying to quit drinking should take three cups of angelica tea every day. To brew the tea, use one teaspoon of angelica and a cup of boiling water. Steep for ten minutes and strain. If you like honey and lemon, add them to taste.

Native Americans used the herb chaparral to heal many ailments. It helps purify the system, ridding the liver of toxins, and easing the urge to drink. Look for chaparral capsules at your local health food store and take one each day to combat alcohol dependency.

Cut Out The Cravings

One of the best ways to curb the appetite for alcohol is to suck on a clove, being careful not to swallow it. Cloves are thought to contain a substance similar to antabuse which short circuits the biochemical pathways that allow alcohol to be broken down efficiently, thus causing discomfort when alcohol is ingested.

Try leaving the liquor out of your next Bloody Mary to break dependence on alcohol. Tart beverages seem to ease alcohol cravings. Take a glass of tomato juice mixed with the juice of a lemon, sipping it slowly.

NEXT-DAY NASTIES: HANGOVER

Prevent The Unpleasantry

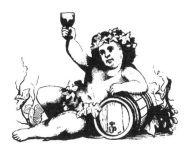

Try eating six raw almonds before you go to the next party to prevent drunkenness. You can also try eating a peanut butter sandwich.

Alcohol acts as a diuretic and depletes the body of needed fluids. It would be wise to drink at least eight ounces of water for every beer and twelve ounces of water for any other alcoholic beverage consumed.

Snacking on raw vegetables and whole grain foods while drinking will usually eliminate a hangover. A number of B vitamins and minerals are needed for the liver to metabolize alcohol. The liver gets overworked and is unable to locate the required nutrients. This depletion is one cause of a hangover.

Take two aspirins with plenty of water before going to bed. This should prevent you from getting a hangover. Don't take aspirin before going out to party or while drinking. It may cause you to get drunker faster.

Sober As A Judge

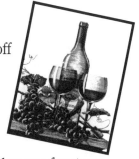

In addition to drinking plenty of water to fight off a hangover, you might also want to include some fruit juice, especially orange juice. The natural sugar helps your body fight off the effects of the alcohol. The vitamin C and potassium also help.

Like fruit juice, honey is also high in the natural sugar fructose, which can speed up the body's ability to burn off alcohol. If you need to sober up in a hurry, take two teaspoons of honey every few minutes, up to two pounds of honey, depending on the amount of alcohol consumed. To cure a hangover, take two tablespoons of honey every minute for five minutes, then do the whole process again thirty minutes later.

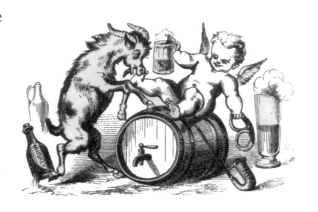

When you've had too much to drink, eat as many cucumber slices as you can. The enzymes in the cucumber will reduce the effects of the alcohol.

Eating certain foods after a night of tying one on really does seem to help cure a hangover. Eat a grapefruit, chewing slowly, to get rid of hangover symptoms. Liquify some fresh radishes in your juicer and drink a small glass. You should sober up quickly.

When You're Feelin' Poorly

"Go sleep it off!" That's common and very good advice when you've had too much to drink. Unfortunately, it may be difficult to follow, since alcohol interferes with your body's natural sleep rhythms. If you wake up the morning after with a hangover, try to nap throughout the day to relieve the symptoms.

The next time you wake up with a nasty headache, sick stomach, and lots of regret, drink a glass of water with an eighth teaspoon cayenne pepper for a quick pick-me-up.

One of the most unpleasant sensations of a hangover is the perception that the room is spinning. It makes you feel more nauseous and can make it difficult to fall asleep. Try lying down on your bed, keeping one foot on the floor to stop the sensation.

Traditional Chinese medicine prescribes ginger tea for the nausea caused by a hangover. You can also stimulate acupressure points to get rid of the other symptoms. To relieve the overall feeling of unwellness, massage the flesh between the thumb and forefinger. Rub each thumb below the knuckle to relieve your pounding headache.

It may sound a little funny, but rub a small piece of lemon, about one quarter of the fruit, under each arm. It will help you feel better after drinking too much.

IT GETS IN YOUR EYES: SMOKING

The Just Say No Remedy

Although in Grandma's day they didn't realize that smoking was harmful, if someone wished to stop smoking she had a remedy that really worked. Place two tablespoons of powdered slippery elm bark into a small mixing bowl. Make a small indentation in the center and pour in a small amount of honey or blackstrap molasses. Mix with the back of a wooden spoon until you have a thick dough. Cut the dough into small pieces and roll them in a mixture of powdered slippery elm bark and a dash of cinnamon for flavor. Suck on one every time you crave a cigarette.

Breaking The Chain

Drinking marjoram tea won't exactly curb your desire to smoke, but it will act as a deterrent (or should I say irritant). Marjoram tea dries the throat, so you won't enjoy those cigarettes quite as much as you have been. Drink the tea straight, you won't need to add a sweetener since marjoram is naturally sweet. In the morning, or when you'd have your first cigarette, drink a half cup. Then, drink a half cup every time you feel a strong urge to smoke.

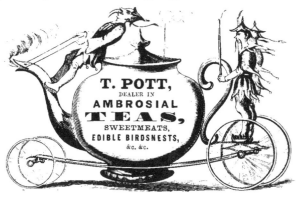

Here's a refreshing alternative to help you stop smoking. Whenever you feel an urge to smoke, eat an orange. But, don't just eat it as you normally would. Try breaking it into sections and eating the pulp after you've sucked out the juice.

Sucking on a clove can eliminate your cigarette craving.

Some people find that a few cups of slipper elm bark tea can curb their desire to smoke. You can buy slippery elm bark tea at most health food stores. Eating a handful of raw, unshelled sunflower seeds can take your mind off of smoking.

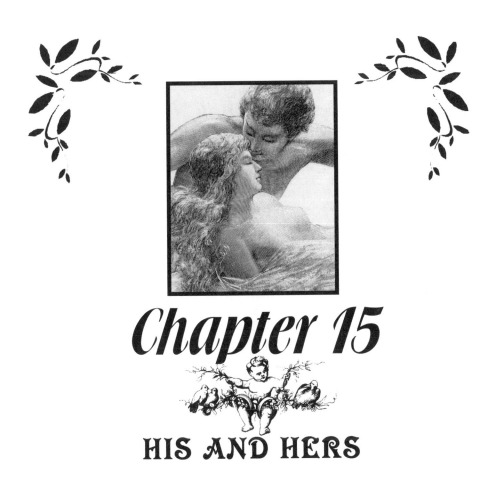

Chapter 15

HIS AND HERS

FEELING FRISKY: APHRODISIAC

Savoy is the most effective herb to increase sexual desire. To prepare the mixture, bring one quart filtered water to a boil and add three and a half tablespoons fenugreek seed. Boil for five minutes. Cover, remove from heat and add eight tablespoons savoy. Steep for one hour and drink two cups before bedtime. The fenugreek acts as a catalyst for the active ingredient in the savoy. Damiana and ginseng are two other herbs that have been used successfully over the years.

HOLDING YOUR NOSE: BODY ODOR

Perspiration is a natural bodily process and should not have an offensive odor. However, if the body needs a cleansing, the sweat glands may pick up toxins and odors from foods that are only partially digested. An herbal cleansing program is recommended in these cases.

From The Inside Out

Try taking zinc supplements, no more than fifteen milligrams a day without a doctor's supervision, to lessen body odor.

Clean out your insides to prevent unpleasant body odor. Fennel tea will do the trick nicely. Create the brew with a teaspoon of dried fennel and a cup of boiled water, steeping for five minutes before straining. Drink the tea first thing in the morning and later in the afternoon. You'll still sweat, but you won't smell a thing and neither will anyone else.

If you have to speak in public or you're going on a job interview and are worried about odor from nervous perspiration, try drinking sage tea. Use one and a half teaspoon of sage to a cup of boiling water, allowing it to set ten minutes before drinking. Drink this tea steadily throughout the day, right up to your big moment.

Common Sense Solutions

Grandma made her own soap, strong stuff, in an old copper kettle. It's not an accident that nobody in her family ever had a problem with body odor. Although my grandmother's recipe is lost to us today, you can buy effective, anti-bacterial soaps such as Dial or Safeguard to help combat body odor.

Chewing a sprig of parsley will cleanse bad breath and may also help reduce body odor. Although it does nothing to stop sweating, the plant's high level of chlorophyll, a natural deodorizer, prevents perspiration from having an unpleasant smell. If you have time to visit your local health food store, look for wheatgrass, another excellent source of chlorophyll. Drink an ounce of wheatgrass a day, always on an empty stomach.

A Sprinkle A Day

Baking soda has been used for many years to combat body odor. Grandma always recommended it to mask unpleasant odors. The baking soda will last longer and be more effective if you make a paste by mixing it with a small amount of water. Placing a small amount in bath water also has an excellent odor controlling quality.

You may not go around craving a glass of fresh radish juice, but it can work wonders on stubborn body odor problems. You can use a juicer, food processor, or blender. It will take several bunches of radishes to make enough juice. Keep it in the refrigerator in a sealed jar. Use it the same way you would an underarm deodorant. You can do the same thing with fresh turnip juice.

Pickling Body Odor

The first time Grandma suggested using apple cider vinegar to relieve body odor, I was skeptical. Personally, I'd rather smell bad than smell like vinegar. But I knew she tended to be right about these things, so I agreed to try it. You don't have to take a bath in it for it to be effective; just dab on a little with a cotton ball. Fortunately, the vinegar smell soon fades, and you feel very clean. Vinegar kills off bacteria that can cause unpleasant odor.

Wash Away The Worry

If you've worked up a sweat digging in your garden or playing with your kids, try taking a warm, relaxing bath, adding a sock filled with fresh mint leaves. The pleasant aroma will relax you, and you'll come out smelling minty fresh.

Use a cucumber wash to deodorize your body naturally. Pick a big, juicy cucumber and cut it into four equal pieces. Rub the slices over the sweaty parts of your body and let your skin air dry. You'll feel fresh and clean as a daisy, and you'll smell just as good.

Dress For Success

According to Grandma, wearing natural fibers reduces the chance of body odor. Since people started dressing in more synthetic clothing, she swears that smelly perspiration problems have greatly increased. It's a fact that natural fibers, like cotton, allow air to circulate more easily, reducing sweating and the possibility of unpleasant body odor.

MOTHER'S MILK: BREAST FEEDING

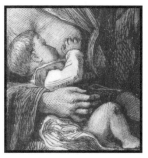

Lactation is a natural, healthful way to feed an infant. Mother's milk is easier to digest, reduces the possibility of allergies to cow's milk, and protects against infections.

When breast feeding, never wash nipples with soap since this will wash away their natural protective coating. Expose them to sunlight and air regularly. Apply aloe vera occasionally to alleviate soreness.

• His And Hers •

Lentils are one of nature's most perfect foods, highly nutritious, full of many vitamins and minerals that are important to the production of breast milk. While nursing your baby, make lentils one of the staples of your diet. Besides, a warm cup of lentil soup is delicious!

Blessed Relief

Many mothers have a problem with breast milk being produced in sufficient quantities. Grandma's cure for this problem was the herb blessed thistle. Make the tea from one to two tablespoons of the dried herb added to one quart boiled water. Allow the mixture to steep for one hour. Strain and drink one cup thirty minutes before nursing.

Peppermint tea is delicious and soothing, helping to settle an upset stomach and relax strained nerves. It can also stimulate lactation and increase the supply of milk.

Traditional folk wisdom tells us that a mixture of fennel and barley water will help increase the supply of breast milk

THE DEEP FREEZE: FRIGIDITY

Frigidity is the inability to experience pleasure or lack of desire for sexual intercourse. It is usually related to an unpleasant experience that has caused psychological fear, or guilt stemming from a childhood event.

A number of herbs, considered to have an aphrodisiac effect, have been used to treat frigidity successfully. They include damiana, ginseng, bee pollen, fo ti and saw palmetto.

Notions From Other Nations

A Middle Eastern remedy for lack of sexual desire is to eat a piece of halvah, made from sesame seeds and honey. Nutrients in the food's ingredients may help stimulate the desire for sex.

Women in France drink a beverage made from powdered licorice and water when they want to pick up the pace in the bedroom. You can find powdered licorice at many health food stores. Add one teaspoon to a cup of water. Licorice contains compounds similar to female hormones that may stimulate the desire for sexual activity.

HERE TODAY, GONE TOMORROW: HAIR LOSS

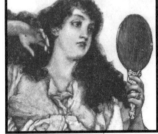

A rinse of sage tea may stimulate hair growth. Saturate a small cloth with the tea and place on the affected areas for fifteen minutes at least four to five times a day.

IF AT FIRST YOU DON'T SUCCEED: IMPOTENCE

Impotence is defined as the inability to achieve or maintain an erection, or premature ejaculation.

Try eating a handful of raw pumpkin seeds each day. The seeds are known to be a sexual stimulant and as an added benefit, can prevent prostate problems.

Diagnosing The Problem

If you suspect that you have this problem, but are not sure, here's a simple test you can perform in your sleep. Buy a roll of postage stamps. Tear off a length of stamps—enough to circle the shaft of the penis. Tape the first and last stamp to each other—careful, don't make it too tight, or too loose. Since most men have about five erections in their sleep, you will be able to tell by morning if your condition is physical or psychological. If you do have an erection during the night, one of the stamp's perforations should tear apart. You might want to try this for several consecutive nights. For some men, just knowing that they achieved an erection at all is enough to relieve the anxiety of trying to have one, and they are then able to achieve an erection while awake.

Herbal Enhancers

A number of herbs have been useful, including gota kola and damiana. You can take them in capsule form or as a tea.

Drinking mint tea can help to restore sexual desire. You can also eat fresh mint leaves. The mint will also make your breath kissably fresh.

The remedy most often recommended by Chinese herbalists is ginseng. The herb comes in many forms, so check your health food store. You should also check with your doctor for the proper dosage before taking the herb.

Garlic is supposed to be excellent for stimulating sexual drive. Add raw garlic to salads, use a lot of garlic in your cooking, and take two garlic pills each day. Besides boosting desire, garlic is supposed to stimulate the production of semen. You might want to follow this garlic remedy with the mint remedy above.

TRY, TRY AGAIN: INFERTILITY

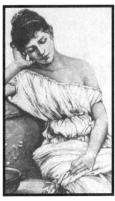

This is the inability to become pregnant or carry a baby to term, usually caused by a hormonal problem.

Take dong quai and gota kola herbs in capsule form.

THE END OF AN ERA: MENOPAUSE

Menopause refers to the point in a woman's life when she stops ovulating. Hormone levels drop and symptoms may include dizziness, headaches, hot flashes, depression and a reduced desire for sexual activity.

Give Your Body What It Needs

The body goes through many changes during menopause, and you may need to supplement your intake of vital nutrients. Make sure you eat a balanced diet. You may also need to take additional B-complex vitamins, calcium and magnesium.

To stop hot flashes, many women take a vitamin E supplement, from 400 to 1,200 milligrams daily, starting at a low dosage and gradually increasing it. You can also get your vitamin E in a multi-vitamin specifically for menopausal women. It's best to check with your doctor before starting a vitamin E regimen.

Restoring The Balance

The herb black cohosh has been used for hundreds of years to reduce the severity of symptoms and seems to have the ability to mimick the effects that estrogen would normally have.

• *His And Hers* •

Suma is an herb that is known for balancing hormones. You can buy this herb in capsule form at most health food stores. Follow the label directions.

A number of other herbs having an effect on the more common symptoms include ginseng, gota kola and dong quai.

Symptom- Reducing Regimens

Make Grandma's morning walk your own habit. Exercise can help reduce the severity of hot flashes or even eliminate them. It will also help ward off heart disease and osteoporosis, two ailments that strike women more commonly after menopause.

To help keep your body temperature at a normal level, drink plenty of water. Try to get eight glasses a day.

Try this breathing exercise to help you get through those hot flashes. Moderate your breathing so that you count to six while breathing in and count to six while breathing out. Breath this way ten times without taking a pause between breaths.

If you feel your face and neck getting flushed, grab an ice cube from the tray, and suck away. The flash will be gone in a flash.

THAT TIME OF THE MONTH: MENSTRUAL PROBLEMS

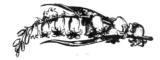 Healing Habits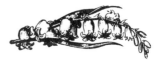

My grandmother prescribed fresh air and exercise for many of life's ills, and she especially recommended a long, relaxing walk, taking the time to listen to the birds and smell the flowers, to relieve menstrual discomfort. Doing some mild exercise while you have your period can help reduce many of the symptoms commonly associated with it, including cramps, bloating and anxiety.

B-complex vitamins appear to be vital in controlling menstrual symptoms. If you have chronic problems, add foods high in B vitamins to your diet, including whole grains, beans, and brewer's yeast. Some women benefit from taking a supplement ten days before the onset of menstruation. These vitamins do a number of things, including regulating estrogen and helping to lessen fatigue and irritability.

To cut down on bloating and cramps, try cutting your salt intake the week before and the week of your period.

Eating leafy green vegetables is a good way to relieve bloating and cramps naturally. Cabbage and a variety of lettuces eaten before and during your period can reduce crampiness and since they are natural diuretics, the vegetables may reduce your bloating. The best way to keep nutrients in cooked vegetables is to steam them. Of course, eating them raw is best, but this may cause gas. Parsley is another good green—so you may want to think twice before you discard this popular restaurant garnish—enjoy.

If you have cramps or lower back pain, nothing feels better than applying heat to the sore muscles, whether from a hot water bottle, heating pad, or warm bath. Heat helps muscles relax, which helps relieve cramps and achiness.

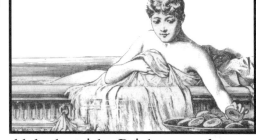

Sweet Relief

For women who have problems with painful menstrual cramps, grandma's remedy should do the trick. Drink a cup of caraway seed tea three times a day, one with each meal. The tea can be made by bringing two to three cups of water to a boil and adding four to five teaspoons of caraway seed that has been made into a powder using a mortar and pestle. After simmering the mixture for five minutes, allow it to steep for approximately fifteen to twenty minutes before drinking. Sweeten with molasses or honey to taste.

For The Natural Woman

A soothing cup of ginger tea will help relieve cramps and an upset stomach. Ginger contains ingredients that reduce pain and fight nausea. You can make a tea by grating fresh ginger root and steeping in hot water for ten minutes. If you can't find fresh ginger, you can also make a tea from two teaspoons ginger powder and one cup boiling water. Many health food stores sell ginger capsules.

The herb dong quai has been used in traditional Chinese medicine to treat gynecological problems for thousands of years. It helps reduce pain, ease bloating, and relax sore, cramping muscles.

This herb is an obvious choice for curbing menstrual cramps: cramp bark. This remedy has been passed down for generations of Native Americans. Beginning the week before your period, drink two cups of cramp bark tea each day. You can find cramp bark tea in many health food stores; it is sometimes called squaw bush.

• His And Hers •

If you have an unusually heavy flow, try drinking yarrow tea. In one cup of boiling water, add one or two teaspoons of dried yarrow. Let the tea steep for ten minutes before straining. Drink two to three cups a day during your period.

There is an herb called suma that has a good reputation for balancing hormones. You can find suma in capsule form at most health food stores—follow the directions on the label.

Off The Wagon

Grandma was a teetotaler, but I heard that she would sip a little warm gin to help relieve her menstrual cramps. Be careful, though. Women who drink right before their period can not only get drunk quicker, but often experience rougher hangovers than they would at other times of the month.

THE MOODY BLUES: PREMENSTRUAL SYNDROME

PMS usually affects women seven to ten days before they begin menstruating. Symptoms are depression, cramps, headaches, breast tenderness, inability to have good sleep patterns, short tempers, and other personality changes.

You Are What You Eat

If you suffer from PMS, you may do well to alter your diet. Reducing your salt intake will help reduce the fluid retention that many women experience. This may be difficult for some, as cravings for salty foods is also a common PMS side-effect.

・ *His And Hers* ・

You may find that avoiding caffeine, sugar and alcohol will also make a difference. These substances are known to affect moods, so if you're prone to moodiness, try eliminating these from your diet (or cutting down)—you'll be pleased with the results.

Increasing calcium intake can be beneficial for easing premenstrual tension and for curbing menstrual cramps. Eat at least one portion of calcium rich foods each day. Some good examples of nutritious foods high in calcium are: leafy greens, including kale, parsley, endive and watercress; and beans, including chickpeas and lentils.

Many women have had success in limiting the effects of PMS by regularly taking B-6 vitamins or B-complex vitamins. Because it is possible to overdo it with vitamins, check with your doctor for his or her recommended dose.

Get A Move On

Many women find that exercise helps reduce many of the side-effects of PMS. Exercise is a vital component of a healthy lifestyle—exercising regularly can reduce stress and increase energy. Many women feel that making it a point to exercise during the week before the beginning of their menstrual cycle alleviates some of their moody swings, lethargy and general lack of energy.

The Herbalist's Checklist

The most effective herbs to alleviate symptoms are dong quai, raspberry leaves, and squaw vine. Either teas, tinctures, or capsules are available in most health food stores.

Chamomile tea is known to do wonders for nerves, so it only makes sense that this tea would be great for premenstrual tension.

237

Make the tea several times throughout the day and sip your PMS away.

Taking two garlic tablets each day can relieve many of the symptoms of PMS including bloating, tender breasts and the blahs.

SIZE MATTERS: PROSTATE PROBLEMS

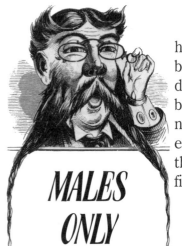

This is one of the most common male health problems. The gland is located beneath the bladder and provides fluids during ejaculation. The gland tends to become enlarged causing difficulty to urinate and is common in older men. Benign enlargement of the gland occurs in over thirty-five percent of men over the age of fifty.

Preventing A Problem

Eating foods rich in vitamin A may ward off prostate problems before they start. Good sources of vitamin A include: leafy green vegetables such as spinach, endive, kale, collard greens and lettuce; broccoli and cauliflower; fish liver oil; carrots; sweet potatoes and winter squash; and fruits such as apricots, papayas, peaches and prunes.

One thing about Peter, Peter, Pumpkin Eater, he probably had a healthy prostate. Eat a handful of raw, shelled, unsalted and unprocessed pumpkin seeds, and you can have one, too. A handful a day should provides vitamins and minerals important for prostate health. (Pumpkin seeds also have a reputation for enhancing sexual drive—maybe Peter was on to something.)

• His And Hers •

Drink one glass of vegetable juice daily. Make the juice from raw asparagus, cucumbers and carrots.

Cucumbers may be beneficial in helping a healthy prostate stay that way. Eat one every day.

Avoid coffee and alcoholic beverages.

Herbal Helpers

The herb saw palmetto taken in capsule form has been known to alleviate the symptoms and may reduce the enlargement.

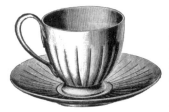

Make a tea from an herb called oatstraw. It should be available in a health food store near you. Add a teaspoon of dried oatstraw to a cup of water that had just boiled. Let steep for ten minutes before drinking.

Soothing Relief

To soothe the prostate area, apply a warm milk compress. Warm up one glass of milk (be careful not to boil) and soak a white towel in it. Place the towel on the area. You may want to cover the compress with a hot water bottle to keep the towel warm longer.

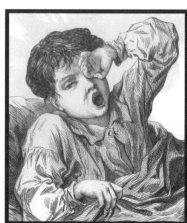

Chapter 16

IT'S ALL IN YOUR HEAD

ABOUT TO DROP: FATIGUE

Wake-Up Call

For those who live in the far north, it can be really hard to get out of bed on a cold winter's day. If you feel tired in the morning and have trouble getting yourself going, combine in a blender two table-spoons apple cider vinegar, one teaspoon honey, and a cup of warm water and blend thoroughly. Drink this liquid wake-up call every morning before breakfast. Within a few days, you should feel like an entirely new person.

If you're mentally exhausted, try this Austrian fatigue-fighter. In a bowl, mix together an unpeeled apple, cut into small pieces, and two cups of boiling water. Let it stand an hour, and then add a tablespoon of honey. Drink the sweetened apple water and eat the apple slices.

To increase your energy, drink a quart of this high power brew a day. Mix six ounces of cranberry juice, all-natural and unsweetened, two ounces of orange juice, and garnish with a fresh lime slice. Add some ice, stir to mix, and enjoy! You'll feel like an Olympic athlete in no time, or at the very least, you'll be able to get out of bed.

High-Energy Health Habits

"If you're tired, go to bed." That was Grandma's hard-to-argue-with logic. Fatigue is the body's natural signal that it needs rest, especially after strenuous physical activity. Take a load off, lie down on the sofa, or spend the day in bed.

On the other hand, too much of a good thing is bad. If you're resting a lot and still feel tired, you may need to get up and go for a walk instead. Grandma took her three-mile walk every morning. She always had plenty of energy and never had trouble sleeping at night.

If the fatigue is not related to an illness, it may be caused by a diet too high in fat and refined carbohydrates, both of which cause sluggishness. Increase your intake of whole grains and fresh fruits and vegetables.

Caffeine and sugar will give you a temporary boost, but you may feel more tired than ever after the effects wear off. To combat that tired feeling from three to five o'clock in the afternoon, make the transition to a caffeine-free life and reduce your sugar intake. After you get used to it, you should feel better than ever.

Vital Herbs

Cayenne increases circulation and may boost energy levels. It may be taken in capsule form. Other useful herbs are ginseng, guarana and gingko biloba.

Revive And Refresh

You know how a hot shower gets you going in the morning? Try a bath or shower to revive whenever you're fatigued. The water will help you feel relaxed and refreshed. In hot weather, cool off by misting yourself with water or splashing cool water on your face.

Nothing could get me out of a deep sleep faster than the smell of bacon frying in Grandma's kitchen. Certain scents seem to have an invigorating effect. Try adding essential oils to your bath, such as peppermint, lavender, or rosemary. For a real kickstart, use a handful of rosemary leaves and lemon rind.

If you find yourself drifting off and need a quick pick-me-up, try this circulation boosting exercise. Press your elbows into your sides or your knees together. It will wake you up, get your blood moving, and make you more mentally alert.

IN OVERDRIVE: HYPERACTIVITY

Hyperactivity has been linked to a disorder of the central nervous system. Symptoms manifest as a lack of concentration, temper tantrums, sleep disorders, and getting easily frustrated when performing a task, among others. It may be linked to artificial preservatives and sweeteners, high consumption of refined carbohydrates, wheat, soft drinks and chocolate.

Take valerian root extract and use according to provided instructions. Valerian root may also be taken in capsule form.

SEARCHING FOR THE SANDMAN: INSOMNIA

Sleeplessness is a serious problem, but it should respond to simple solutions. It may be caused by a variety of drugs, low blood sugar, asthma, stress, or even a lack of certain minerals such as calcium and magnesium.

Sweet Dreams Diet Plan

The mineral magnesium, with its muscle relaxing properties, can help you get to sleep more readily. Two hours before bedtime, take 400 milligrams of magnesium, along with 50 milligrams of vitamin B6 to facilitate the body's use of magnesium. Of course, you should always check with your doctor before taking any supplements.

Eating lots of lettuce late in the evening may help you get a more restful night's sleep. But, be aware that lettuce acts as a diuretic, so while it may relax you so you can fall asleep, it may also wake you so you can go to the bathroom.

• *It's All In Your Head* •

Eliminating salt from your evening meal can help prevent sleep-lessness. So can cutting out after-dinner snacks. In fact, it is recom-mended that you have your last meal several hours before you turn in for the night.

Goat's milk has been known to help some insomniacs get some zzzzs. Try drinking six ounces of goat's milk before each meal and another six ounces before bedtime. Some peo-ple have reported a better night's sleep within a week. Goat's milk is available in some health food stores.

Rest For The Weary

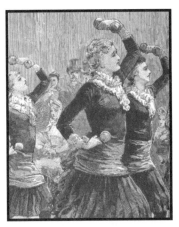

This is a remedy for insomnia that has a host of excellent side effects. Exercise. Be sure to exercise regularly but be sure to workout during the day—never before bedtime. The extra energy will just keep you awake.

If you have young children, you know how letting them run around like crazy, playing as hard as they can during the day, tires them out so they can get a good night's sleep. We're not so different from our kids. Getting exercise or doing hard physical work will wear you out, and you'll have no problem drifting off.

Grandma always stretched and did her deep breathing exercises before turning in for the night. It was part of her usual routine. Stretching aids circulation which promotes restfulness. Concentrate on slowing down your breath to help you relax.

Bedtime Rituals

Grandma always said counting sheep just made the sheep tired. Here's a remedy for the rest of us who don't feel like jumping over fences all night long. Try taking a warm bath in the evening. Add some aromatic oils that you can buy in a health food store. Many boutiques also sell aromatherapy oils. Make sure you buy the kind that are good for relaxation. While soaking, sip some herbal tea such as chamomile, ginger or Celestial Seasoning's Sleepy Time Tea. You might also try reading a book or lighting some candles. You should feel relaxed (and pampered). Make sure you head right to bed, and snuggle in for a good night's sleep.

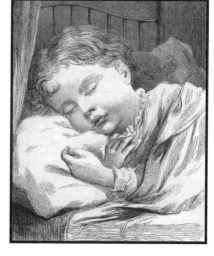

One home remedy that just about everyone has heard of is warm milk. It's been around forever, and there's a good reason: it works. Grandma swore by this. She would enjoy a cup of warm milk almost every night. And, like everything else she did, Grandma would jazz it up a bit. She would add honey to taste (about one or two teaspoons should do) and a half teaspoon of nutmeg. Then, she would sit quietly and sip, relax and enjoy.

Remember how hard it was to keep your eyes open in math class in the late afternoon? Or how riding in a car or on a train will put you right out? If you have a hard time falling asleep, try boring yourself into unconsciousness. Read a book before turning in or recite a poem in your head, whatever will distract you from thinking about how much you want to go to sleep and how badly you need the rest. These relaxing pastimes should help relax you and lull you to sleep.

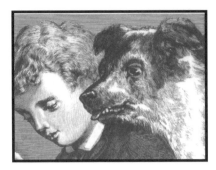

Snuggling Up

If you love animals, try having your pets sleep in the same bed with you. It's been shown that pets help people relax and can actually lower blood pressure. If you wake up in the middle of the night and have trouble getting back to sleep, pet your cat or dog. It will quiet you and hopefully make you feel drowsy again.

Calm In A Cup

The most effective herb is valerian root, taken in capsule form or as a tea. Certain foods that have a high level of tryptophan promote sleep. They include tuna, bananas, turkey and dates. This is why you get tired after Thanksgiving dinner.

The herbs passionflower and hops help reduce anxieties and tension that may prevent you from getting a good night's sleep. Take these herbs powdered in capsules or brew into a tea. To a lesser degree, chamomile and sage also act as sleep aids. Use these remedies to help with occasional sleeplessness. You should not rely upon them to help you fall asleep on a regular basis.

Catnip For A Cat Nap

I once saw grandma mixing up a concoction made from catnip. At the time, I thought that she was making a special treat for our cats. To my surprise, she gave the tea to my grandfather who had been complaining of insomnia. It seems catnip contains a chemical called nepelactone which is biochemically similar to a chemical in valerian root. A cup of catnip tea at bedtime should guarantee a naturally good night's sleep.

246

The Better Part Of Valor

Sometimes the best answer is just not to fight it. If you can't sleep, get up and do something. Pay bills, catch up on paperwork or letterwriting, find out what's showing on the late show. You will sleep when you get tired enough. Usually a couple of days as a night owl is enough to cure sleeplessness.

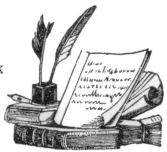

IQ INVASION: MEMORY PROBLEMS

Food For Thought

Diets that are high in processed low nutrition foods tend to cause a reduction in mental powers. Consume more natural raw foods, especially whole grains high in Vitamin B.

Deficiency of Vitamin B12 has been linked to nervous system problems and impairment of mental facilities. Older people are especially prone to this vitamin deficiency. Check with your doctor to see if this may be a problem for you and what an appropriate dosage is.

Eating raw almonds each day can help to improve your memory. Nuts are very high in fat, so only a few (five or six) should do the trick. Sunflower seeds can do the trick, too. Just a handful a day is all you'll need.

Same Time, Same Place

Memory is context specific. Clinical studies have shown that college students who study in the same place and at the same time of day that an exam is given do significantly better than those who study elsewhere and at other times of day. If you learn something in a particular environment, returning to those conditions makes it easier to remember.

You can put the psychologists' research to work in your own life. If you're studying for a test or just trying to keep a grip on what you have to do this week, try adding a scent to it. Study or go over your schedule while breathing in a distinctive fragrance—lavender, cinnamon, rosemary, or anything else that appeals to you. Whenever you need to jolt your memory, take a whiff of the scent.

Rescue Your Recall

The herb gota kola has been used to increase memory effectiveness for hundreds of years. You should be able to find capsules at your local health food store.

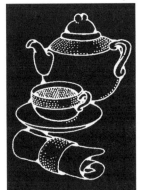

An herb called yerba mate has a lot of fans who claim that among other fine qualities, this herb helps to increase memory. Try it for yourself. Drink one cup each morning. But, be aware that unlike most herb teas, this one contains caffeine (although it does contain less caffeine than coffee).

Eyebright tea can boost your memory. To one and a half cups of boiling water add a half ounce of eyebright and one tablespoon of clover honey. Let steep until cool. Strain and put in a container. Drink three quarters cup of the tea before lunch and dinner.

Make sage tea and add three or four cloves. This combination is supposed to strengthen the memory. You can drink this tea once a day.

Picking Up The Scent

Why not try aromatherapy to improve your memory? Smelling crushed caraway seeds can help sharpen your recollection. You can also try ground cloves or coriander seeds.

BRIGHT-EYED AND BUSHY-TAILED: MENTAL ALERTNESS

For physical as well as mental energy, try bee pollen. After breakfast, take one teaspoon of granular pollen, or if you prefer, take two 500 mg pollen pills. Many people notice a difference in alertness and memory within weeks of first taking the pollen.

Another very effective method of increasing mental alertness and improving memory is to consume one to two teaspoons of Brazil nut powder in a cup of juice. There are specific amino acids that stimulate brain function found in the Brazil nut.

What Did You Say That Cure Was?

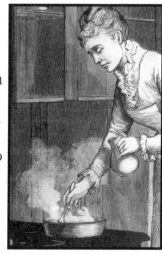

Whenever someone in my family had a problem remembering, Grandma would go looking for a fresh artichoke. She would pull the artichoke leaves off and place them into a jar with just enough water to cover the leaves. She would then place the jar in a pan of water and bring it to a boil allowing the jar to remain in the boiling water for at least two hours. As the water boiled away, she kept adding more so that the boiling water was up to the level of the solution in the jar. She would then strain the contents and squeeze

249

the leaves until all the liquid was removed. She would then have the forgetful one take three tablespoons of this artichoke broth, three to four times a day for five days. Once again, Grandma knew best: Studies have shown that artichoke leaves contain substances similar in nature to caffeine.

BYE, BYE BUTTERFLIES: NERVOUSNESS

Kiss It Goodbye

If you are prone to nervousness, you should cut caffeine out of your diet. Besides tea, coffee and colas, you should avoid chocolate. Substitute herbal teas for the caffeinated beverages and carob for chocolate. Carob is available in many varieties in health food stores. It has the consistency of chocolate and is used in all of the same ways. Carob treats should curb your chocolate craving without adding caffeine to your diet.

Tranquilizing Tonics

The remedy for nervousness and hyperactivity are basically the same, celery juice. Both the stalk and the seeds of celery contain the substance "phthalide." Since raw celery juice is not very appealing, you might want to add a small amount of honey to sweeten it. Consume a quarter cup daily for about three days to solve the problem. Celery juice has also been used successfully to lower blood pressure.

Drink sage tea three times a day. You can buy sage tea bags at your health food store. If you prefer to use dry herbs, use one teaspoon to one cup of warm water. Let steep for several minutes.

Foods That Fight Stress

A seaweed called kombu is said to make an excellent tea for nerves. Kombu and other seaweed is readily available at health food stores. In a quart of water, boil a three-inch strip of the kombu for ten minutes. Drink the tea throughout the day in a half cup portions.

Onions are said to have a relaxing quality. Finely chop one large onion into tiny pieces and mix in one tablespoon of honey. Eat half of the onion mixture with lunch, and half with dinner.

If you have a sudden stressful situation occur, try eating a handful of sesame seeds. They're rich in calcium and can help you get through the emotional episode.

Eating strawberries in season can calm your nerves. Just a few berries after each meal is a great, relaxing treat.

Kicking Back

Try taking a relaxing Epsom salt bath—Grandma swore by them. Pour two cups of Epsom salt into your warm bath. Soak for half an hour and feel the tension drain from you. Dim the lights for even more relaxation.

Listening to calming music may just do the trick, especially if your tension stems from a difficult day at the office. You might try combining this with the cure above and bring the radio into the bathroom.

FORGET ME NOT: SENILITY

This lessening of mental powers and memory often occurs in the elderly, and may be caused by the increase in medications taken by this age group.

The herb gingko biloba has been used effectively in capsule form as well as gota kola. A combination of blue cohosh and anise has also been effective.

THE END OF YOUR ROPE: STRESS

Valerian root capsules have produced excellent results in reducing stress and anxiety levels. Teas made from chamomile and pau d'arco are also very effective.

Low Stress Lifestyle

One of the simplest answers to stress is something my grandmother always said: "Take time to enjoy life!" Have more fun, whatever that means for you. Get out of the house and get some exercise, a quieting walk like my grandmother enjoyed. Pet owners are less likely to suffer from stress-related disorders, so consider adopting a cat or dog. Take time every day for yourself, to meditate or nap or just have a few quiet moments alone.

A number of foods tend to aggravate a stressful condition and should be avoided. These include sugars, fried foods, colas, products containing white flour and potato chips.

When You're Under The Gun

When anxiety attacks, focus on your breathing, slowing it down, inhaling more deeply, and exhaling fully. It will help calm down other stress symptoms, such as racing heart beat and tense muscles.

Traditional healing recognizes the ability of certain scents
to effect changes in the body. Using essential oils like
lavender, rosemary, and pine in your bath can help relax
muscles and relieve stress. Try putting pots of apple-cinna-
mon potpourri around your house to make your home a low-
stress zone.

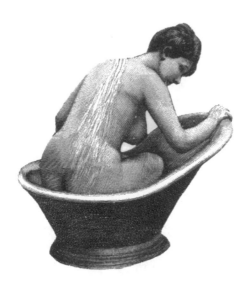

When you're feeling pressure, think acupressure.
Massage the webbed area on your left hand between the thumb and
index finger. Really work on it, kneading for five minutes—it will
probably hurt. After a while, you'll notice that the pain will decrease,
and so will your tension.

Draw yourself a warm bath, add some bubbles, and settle in for a
long soak. Create a sensual get-away for yourself by lighting candles
and playing soothing music. Use your imagination to leave worries
behind you. Picture yourself on a tropical island, floating in warm,
clear, blue-green water. By the time you get out of the tub, you
won't remember why you were stressed out in the first place.

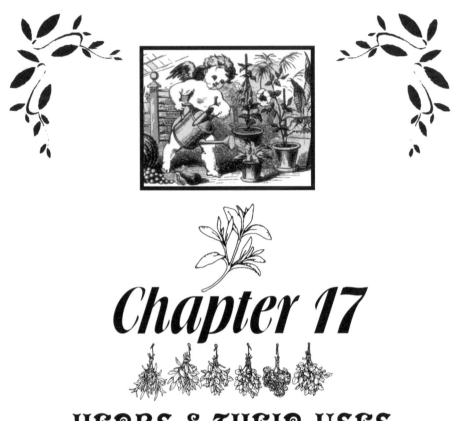

Chapter 17

HERBS & THEIR USES

Below is a list of herbs and spices, many of which Grandma grew and used for her home remedies. It's important to remember that, as with all medicines, you should check with a doctor before undertaking any herbal remedy. Some herbs are toxic if taken at the wrong dosage. Some should only be used topically. Others may cause skin irritation, block the body's proper absorption of vital nutrients, or interact dangerously with other herbs or medications you are taking. Certain herbs should never be taken by pregnant or lactating women, and these women should be especially careful to consult a physician before starting any herbal therapy. Of course, the same is true for giving herbs or any other medication to children. Individuals may be sensitive to certain substances. You should take all necessary precautions, including doing a patch test, to check for allergic reactions before using any herb.

Poultice

A poultice is normally made from a relatively soft, moist mixture of herbs and other compounds or oils. It is prepared in a paste form and usually spread between two very thin pieces of cloth or thin dishtowels. This is then placed on the area of the body that is affected. Poultices normally are used to increase blood flow, soothe injured tissues, relax muscles that have become tense or strained, and may be used to draw toxins from injured areas.

Most poultices are prepared from dried herbs using a mortar and pestle to powder the herbs. The herbs are placed into a glass or ceramic bowl and sufficient filtered water added to make a paste that can be easily used.

Using a clean piece of cloth large enough to cover the affected area, evenly spread the paste over the surface of the cloth. The area should first be cleansed with hydrogen peroxide before applying the poultice. After applying the poultice place another cloth over the poultice and wrap to avoid any of the paste getting on clothing.

The period of time to leave a poultice on will vary depending on the type of injury. Poultices may be left on for a few hours to a full day in some instances. Fresh poultices may be applied at regular intervals as needed. An occasional throbbing pain may mean that the poultice is working to draw out infection and should subside in a short period of time.

Be sure and wash the area thoroughly after removing the poultice. Irritating herbs such as mustard should never be placed directly on the skin but placed between two pieces of cloth. Herbs used should be as fresh as possible to be effective.

Alfalfa

A perennial herb grown throughout the world in various climates, the leaves of the alfalfa plant are rich in nutrients and minerals. It is also recognized as an excellent source of chlorophyll and vitamins.

Common uses include:

- Arthritis
- Blurred vision
- Edema
- Hay Fever
- Indigestion
- Infections

Allspice

Grown primarily in Jamaica, allspice was first brought to Europe by Christopher Columbus. It gets its common name from its flavor—a combination of the spices, cloves, cinnamon and nutmeg. It's a versatile spice that can be used in both sweet and savory cooking.

Common uses include:

- Diarrhea

Aloe Vera

Another name for this versatile healer is "medicine plant." Known as a moisturizer, skin softener and skin healer, aloe vera is used in many cosmetic and hair products. Use of this plant to heal burns dates back to ancient Egypt. A hearty plant, there are hundreds of different species that grow in dry regions around the world.

Common uses include:

- Age spots
- Burns
- Cold Sores
- Facial Swelling
- Flatulence
- Hemorrhoids
- Shingles
- Sunburn
- Toothache
- Ulcers

Angelica

Believed to have been named for the Archangel Raphael, angelica is one of nature's most versatile herbs.

Common uses include:

- Alcohol Dependency
- Headaches

Anise

Anise seed has a sweet flavor, similar to licorice. It is a good natural sweetener often used to flavor toothpaste and other mouthwash and breath freshening products. Anise is good for digestion.

Common uses include:

- Bad Breath
- Flatulence
- Hoarseness
- Indigestion
- Senility

Arnica

Commonly called "leopard's bane," the arnica plant produces bright yellow flowers each July. Homeopathic medicines have been produced from its daisy-like flowers for hundreds of years.

Common uses include:

- Muscle Stiffness
- Varicose Veins

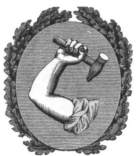

Arrowroot

A tropical plant whose roots are used to make starches used in baking and other culinary purposes. It's most common use is in teething biscuits for children.

Common uses include:

- Bruises
- Indigestion

Astragalus

This is one of the most famous herbs used in traditional Chinese medicine. Its use dates back to the first century. According to Chinese herbalists, this herb is good for strengthening the body's vital energy. It is used in many common ailments.

Common uses include:

- Immune System

Barberry Bark

Also known as bayberry, this native American plant is one of the most versatile herbs. It was often prescribed by 19th century physicians. It is an expectorant and is frequently used in mouthwash.

Common uses include:

- Constipation
- Hyperthyroid
- Varicose Veins
- Gallbladder Problems
- Ulcers

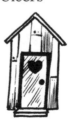

Basil

You may think of basil as a favorite ingredient in tomato sauce, but in fact, basil has been used for its healing abilities since the sixth century. This is a delicious herb that is used as an effective remedy for a variety of symptoms.

Common uses include:

- Arthritis
- Headache

Bee Pollen

Sometimes called "nature's perfect food," bee pollen is very rich in vitamins minerals and amino acids including B-complex vitamins, vitamin C, vitamin D, vitamin E, carotene, calcium, lecithin, magnesium and protein.

Common uses include:

- Frigidity
- Hay Fever
- Mental Alertness
- Physical Energy

Birch Bark

Birch Bark contains vitamins A, C, B1, B2 and E, as well as calcium, chlorine, iron, potassium and other minerals. This herb has been used for a number of ailments.

Common uses include:

- Eczema

Black Cohosh

This root has long been used by Native Americans to treat "female problems."

Common uses include:

- Hyperthyroid
- Menopause

Blessed Thistle

Blessed thistle is often used in commercial herbal preparations designed for use by women.

Common uses include:

- Breast Feeding

Blueberry Leaf

Blueberry leaf is an antiseptic and an astringent. It has several different uses in folk medicine.

Common uses include:

- Blue Cohosh
- Diabetes

Although many advise against using this herb while pregnant, Native American Indian women used to drink a tea made from this herb to help ease the birth process. You may find blue cohosh effective for a number of different symptoms.

Common uses include:

- Senility

Burdock

Natural healers have been using this herb for centuries. Ancient herbalists are said to have used burdock for snake bites.

Common uses include:

• Headache

Calendula

Calendula contains vitamin A, vitamin C and phosphorus. Often used as an astringent, it is considered an excellent first aid remedy.

Common uses include:

• Varicose Veins

Camphor

For hundreds of years, camphor has been distilled from the wood of the camphor tree. It's use dates back to the 12th century.

Common uses include:

• Cold Sores

Caraway Seed

These aromatic seeds come from an herb in the parsley family. The seeds are used to flavor many foods including breads, cheese, vegetables and stews.

Common uses include:

• Colic
• Indigestion

• Memory Problems
• Menstrual Problems

Cardamom

A member of the ginger family, this aromatic spice is native to India and is used in many East Indian dishes.

Common uses include:

- Indigestion

Cat Nip

You may already be using cat nip for your felines, but this aptly named herb has some beneficial qualities for humans, too.

Common uses include:

- Flu
- Gallbladder Problems
- Insomnia
- Measles and Mumps
- Ulcers

Cayenne Pepper

You may not care for spicy foods, but research has shown that they can care for you—if they're spiced with cayenne, that is. Cayenne is very nutritious and has been found to have many beneficial qualities for curing a number of ailments.

Common uses include:

- Artery Health Test
- Arthritis
- Bleeding
- Colds
- Cold Hands
- Cold Feet
- Cuts and Scrapes
- Diarrhea
- Headache
- High Blood Pressure
- Indigestion
- Motion Illness
- Muscle Stiffness
- Nosebleeds
- Sore Throat
- Toothache
- Ulcers

Chamomile

One of the most well-known herbs, nearly everyone has heard of or tried chamomile tea at one time or another. Chamomile is known for its calming effect, it also has a number of external benefits. Chamomile is added to many shampoos to enhance blond highlights.

Common uses include:

- Dandruff
- Diarrhea
- Eye Problems
- Flatulence
- Hay Fever
- High Blood Pressure
- Indigestion
- Insomnia
- Muscle Stiffness
- Nausea
- Oily Skin
- Premenstrual Syndrome
- Sore Throat
- Stress
- Toothache
- Ulcers

Chaparral

This North American plant was used by Native Americans. It is useful for a number of ailments.

Common uses include:

- Alcohol Dependency
- Psoriasis
- Skin Solution
- Worms

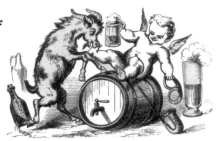

Chervil

Chervil is a mild-flavored member of the parsley family. Although chervil is used mostly for its leaves, early Greeks and Romans were said to enjoy the root.

Common uses include:

- Eye Problems

Chickweed

This herb has been found useful in folk medicine for a number of ailments.

Common uses include:

• Itching

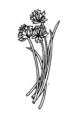

Chive

This herb is related to the onion and leek. Chives are a good source of vitamin A and also contain some potassium and calcium.

Common uses include:

• Dandruff

Cinnamon

This is an aromatic spice valued for its use in both savory and sweet cooking. In ancient times, cinnamon was used to treat a number of ailments including colds, menstrual cramps and for flatulence.

Common uses include:

• Bad Breath   • Diarrhea   • Nausea
• Bed Wetting   • Flu   • Smoking
• Cold   • Memory Problems   • Stress
• Cough

Cleavers

Cleavers has a number of uses in both cosmetic and health care. Used as an infusion, it is said to be good for the complexion and is helpful as a hair rinse for dandruff. It is also used as a natural deodorant.

Common uses include:

- Weight Control
- Wrinkles

Clove

It is said that during the Han dynasty anyone who addressed the Chinese emperor was required to hold cloves in their mouths to mask their bad breath. Clove was also brought back to Spain by Magellan in 1512 when the explorer finished his first voyage around the world. It has many uses both culinary and medicinal.

Common uses include:

- Alcohol Dependency
- Arthritis
- Asthma
- Bad Breath
- Cold Sores
- Constipation
- Cough
- Diarrhea
- Gout
- Hay fever
- Hemorrhoids
- High blood pressure
- Inflammation
- Kidney problems
- Memory problems
- Nausea
- Smoking
- Sore Throat
- Toothache

Comfrey

Both the root and leaves of this plant are used by herbal healers. The root is said to be useful for skin wounds, while the leaves are traditionally thought to be good for blood cleansing and strengthening.

Common uses include:

- Black eyes
- Bruises
- Burns
- Snakebite

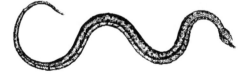

Cornsilk

For many years, cornsilk has been used for a variety of ailments including bedwetting and urinary tract ailments.

Common uses include:

- Arthritis
- Bladder infections

Cramp Bark

Cramp bark is high in vitamins C and K, potassium, calcium and magnesium.

Common uses include:

- Menstrual cramps

Damiana

This plant has been rumored to be good for jump starting sexual desire, most likely because its Latin name sounds suspiciously like the word aphrodisiac. In truth, it is considered a good nerve tonic.

Common uses include:

- Aphrodisiac
- Frigidity
- Impotence

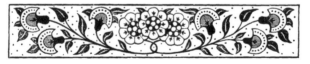

Dandelion

Although you may think of dandelion as a hearty weed plaguing your garden, dandelion has a number of beneficial qualities. It is rich in potassium and lecithin—substances that are beneficial for healthy bodies.

Common uses include:

- Diabetes
- Edema
- Gall bladder problems
- Gout
- Liver cleansing
- Warts

Dill

Both the leaves and seeds of this plant are used as condiments.

Common uses include:

- Cough
- Hiccups

Dong Quai

Grown in Japan, China and Korea, this herb is rich in vitamins and minerals and is said to possess properties similar to ginseng as an "all-purpose" tonic for women.

Common uses include:

- Infertility
- Menopause
- Menstrual Problems
- Premenstrual Syndrome

Echinacea

This North American perennial has become very popular in many health store cold and flu preparations over the last few years.

Common uses include:

- Flu
- Inflammation
- Mumps

Elderberry

You may know elderberry as a kind of wine, pie or jam, but this herb was used for its healing properties by many early American Indian tribes. It is a good source of vitamin A, vitamin B and vitamin C.

Common uses include:

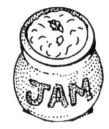

• Coughs

Eucalyptus

Eucalyptus has a strong medicinal smell that helps to clear breathing passages. It is a natural antiseptic, antibiotic, antiviral, diuretic, analgesic and anti-inflammatory agent.

Common uses include:

• Arthritis	• Colds	• Cough
• Athlete's Foot	• Congestion	• Sinusitis

Eyebright

This herb has been used as a tonic and an astringent since the Middle Ages.

Common uses include:

• Eye Problems	• Memory Problems

Fennel

Used for centuries, fennel is a spice that can be put to many uses—both culinary and medicinal.

• Herbs & Their Uses •

Common uses include:

- Body Odors
- Breast Feeding
- Colic
- Eye Problems
- Flatulence
- Flu
- Gallbladder
- Indigestion
- Weight Control

Fenugreek

This is one of the oldest medicinal plants; its use dates back to the ancient Egyptians.

Common uses include:

- Aphrodisiac
- Cough
- Ears, Ringing
- Hay Fever
- Indigestion

Feverfew

Feverfew is regarded as a valuable treatment of migraine headaches and some of their side effects.

Common uses include:

- Migraine

Flaxseed

Flaxseed oil is one of nature's richest sources of essential fatty acids. It is effective in the treatment and prevention of many ailments.

Common uses include:

- Constipation
- High Blood Pressure
- Itching
- Kidney Problems
- Muscle Stiffness

269

Fo ti

The Chinese use this for a "rejuvenating tonic" and believe it can prevent certain signs of aging.

Common uses include:

• Frigidity

Garlic

Although Count Dracula may disagree, garlic is one of the most popular culinary herbs. It is also regarded as one of the most valuable foods on the planet. Used since biblical times, garlic is an effective remedy for a wide range of ailments.

Common uses include:

• Arthritis	• Ear Infection	• Impotence
• Asthma	• Edema	• Insect Bites
• Athlete's Foot	• Flatulence	• Kidney Infections
• Bedsores	• Fungus	• Measles
• Bladder Infections	• Gout	• Premenstrual Syndrome
• Colds	• Headache	• Sinusitis
• Cold Sores	• Hemorrhoids	• Skin Solutions
• Cough	• High Blood Pressure	• Smoking
• Diabetes	• High Cholesterol	• Sore Throat
• Diarrhea	• Immune System	• Warts

Ginger

Many cooks know what ginger can do for a main dish or dessert, but this herb has been used for over two thousand years by Asian herbalists.

• Herbs & Their Uses •

Common uses include:

- Arthritis
- Asthma
- Charley Horse
- Cold
- Cold Feet
- Colic
- Congestion
- Cough
- Dandruff
- Diarrhea
- Eye Problems
- Flatulence
- Flu
- Food Poisoning
- Frostbite
- Heartburn
- Insomnia
- Menstrual Cramps
- Motion Illness
- Muscle Stiffness
- Nausea
- Pneumonia
- Sore Throat
- Ulcers

Ginko Biloba

This is a strong herb that is believed to have many positive effects on brain function.

Common uses include:

- Migraine

Ginseng

This popular healing herb has many uses. There are many types of ginseng including American, Chinese, Korean and Japanese varieties.

Common uses include:

- Aphrodisiac
- Asthma
- Diabetes
- Fatigue
- Frigidity
- Impotence
- Memory Problems
- Menopause

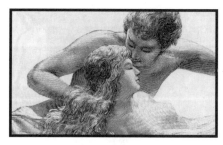

Goldenseal

This North American plant, belonging to the buttercup family, has long been a staple of traditional healing. It was used by Native Americans for medicinal purposes, but also as a yellow dye for cloth and other materials.

Common uses include:

- Colds
- Constipation
- Cuts and scrapes
- Dermatitis
- Eye problems
- Flu
- Headaches
- High cholesterol
- Hyperthyroid
- Inflammation
- Pneumonia
- Poison ivy and oak
- Psoriasis

Gota kola

This herb was first put into practice in India and has been used in Chinese medicine for two thousand years. It has become increasingly popular in the West during the past few years. According to Asian healers, gota kola revives energy levels and strengthens the nervous system. They sometimes refer to it as "brain food."

Common uses include:

- Age spots
- Impotence
- Infertility
- Memory problems
- Menopause
- Senility

Grape vine leaves

These leaves are used in certain dishes in Middle Eastern cuisine. They also have some medicinal applications.

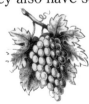

Common uses include:

- Hemorrhoids

Guarana

This climbing shrub is native to South America. Its seeds are harvested and ground into a powder that is somewhat similar to cocoa. Brazilian miners drink a beverage made from it and believe it is effective in preventing many illnesses.

Common uses include:

• Fatigue

Hops

This plant was used as far back as the ancient Romans. It has a wide variety of uses. The herb is most well-known for its role in the brewing of beer. However, it can also be eaten as a vegetable. The tough fibers of its stem have been used to produce a coarse and durable cloth, and the leaves yield a brown dye.

Common uses include:

• Insomnia   • Nervousness   • Stress

Horehound

This herb is widely used in making tea and candy. The bushy plant thrives in scrub areas, in ditches and along the sides of roads. For thousands of years, it has been highly valued for its medicinal properties, and was used by the ancient Egyptians, Hebrews, and Romans. An effective expectorant, it is an ingredient in some commercial cough syrups and lozenges.

Common uses include:

• Colds   • Coughs   • Weight control

Horseradish

A great compliment to roast beef when sliced thin and mixed with a little vinegar, this root can also be powerful medicine. Horseradish has been grown from the earliest ages and was greatly valued for its therapeutic properties during the Middle Ages. It is a strong diuretic.

Common uses include:

- Arthritis
- Asthma
- Colds
- Coughs
- Frostbite
- Hay fever
- Headaches
- Sinusitis

Horsetail

This herb is an effective diuretic and astringent. It grows in the wild in shady and moist environments, often along the banks of rivers and streams.

Common uses include:

- Bloodshot eyes
- Nail problems

Hyssop

Its common name comes from the Greek and refers to the fact that it was used to clean sacred places such as temples. This bushy evergreen herb is cultivated for its flowertops, which have both medicinal and culinary value. In the kitchen, it can be put into broths and salads. Some varieties are also used to make liqueurs and perfume. It is well-known as an expectorant.

Common uses include:

- Colds
- Colitis
- Constipation
- Coughs
- Gout
- Headaches
- Hemorrhoids
- High blood pressure
- Sore throats

Jewelweed

This plant is also known as impatiens or touch-me-nots. Its blossoms come in many colors—red, pink, white, yellow, and purple. The herb has a variety of uses, many medicinal ones, and the flowers produce a yellow dye.

Common uses include:

- Poison ivy and oak
- Rash

Juniper

A 16th century Dutch pharmacist, looking for an effective and inexpensive diuretic, turned juniper berries into a beverage that remains popular to our day—gin. For hundreds of years, juniper has been used in folk remedies for a variety of ailments.

Common uses include:

- Gout
- Infections

Kelp

This variety of seaweed is highly nutritious, a rich source of vitamins, especially B-complex, and minerals. Kelp is eaten raw in Japan, but can also be found in powdered or liquid form, as well as tablets and capsules.

Common uses include:

- Arthritis
- Bleeding
- Edema
- High blood pressure
- Indigestion

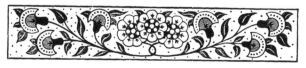

Kombu

This variety of seaweed is an essential ingredient in one of Japanese cooking's staple stocks. Like all seaweed, it is highly nutritious, containing a variety of vitamins and minerals.

Common uses include:

- Nervousness
- Stress

Laurel (bay leaf)

In Greek mythology, this plant was sacred to Apollo. Wreaths of its leaves decorated the heads of heroes and triumphant athletes in ancient Greece and Rome. The herb is most commonly used in cooking. It can also be used in the production of perfume.

Common uses include:

- Colds
- Dandruff
- Coughs
- Flatulence

Lavender

Best known for its lovely scent, this herb graces many gardens. It is widely used in soaps, perfumes, air fresheners, and potpourri. Sachets containing lavender are often placed in drawers to protect clothing from moths. However, the oil extracted from lavender flowers has many medicinal uses as well.

Common uses include:

- Fatigue
- High blood pressure
- Skin problems
- Hay fever
- Memory problems
- Stress

Ledum

Herbalists have used this plant for some medicinal purposes.

Common uses include:

• Bruises

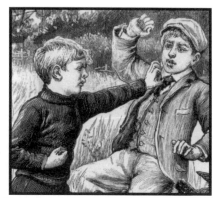

Lemon Balm

In the kitchen, this herb flavors beverages, fish and cheese dishes. It has a lovely scent, and the essential oil is used in aromatherapy as a pick-me-up and to treat depression. Herbalists prescribe an infusion of lemon balm for a variety of ailments.

Common uses include:

• Depression (aromatherapy)   • Fevers

Licorice

Many of us are familiar with licorice exclusively as a flavoring for candy and liqueurs, however this herb has valuable medicinal applications as well. Traditional healers use it to treat illnesses involving the upper respiratory tract. It is an effective expectorant.

Common uses include:

• Asthma   • Coughs   • Sore throats
• Bad breath   • Frigidity   • Ulcers
• Colds   • Oily skin

Lobelia

Named after the botanist Matthias de Lobel, this herb has been used in a wide variety of ways by many different communities, including Native Americans and colonists who settled in New England.

Common uses include:

- Ear infections
- Fevers
- Headaches
- Measles
- Mumps

Marjoram

This herb is valued primarily for its culinary applications. It is aromatic, similar to basil and fennel. The oil extracted from its leaves also has medicinal uses.

Common uses include:

- Heartburn
- Motion sickness
- Indigestion
- Smoking

Marshmallow

The white, sticky food available at your local supermarket does not contain this herb as an ingredient, although it is sometimes used in other confections. Known for thousands of years for its healthful properties, marshmallow gets its name from a Greek word which means "to cure." It has many applications. The plant has been eaten as a vegetable by the Egyptians, Romans, Chinese, and other peoples. Medicinally, it has laxative and emollient properties.

Common uses include:

- Edema
- Kidney problems

Mugwort

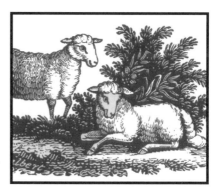

Said to take its name from its use in flavoring drinks, this herb was used in the brewing of beer before hops took its place. It is found abundantly in the wild. Tradition has it that it is useful in fattening sheep and poultry.

Common uses include:

- Poison Ivy and Oak
- Rashes

Mullein

This weed is also commonly known as golden rod and can be found growing wild in many locations, especially on the east coast. From ancient times, mullein tea has been used to treat a wide variety of ailments, most especially upper respiratory tract problems.

Common uses include:

- Asthma
- Colds
- Coughs
- Hay fever
- Sore throat

Myrrh

One of the gifts brought by the three wise men, this herb has long been used as a main ingredient in perfume, holy oil, and incense. The ancient Egyptians also appear to have employed it for embalming. It has a number of healing applications as well.

Common uses include:

- Bad breath
- Canker sores
- Body odor
- Cold sores

Nettles

It may seem unlikely that this stinging plant would have health benefits, but in fact, it is a rich source of vitamins and minerals, especially vitamin C. It can be prepared and eaten like spinach or made into a soup or tea. This herb has traditionally been used in a number of medicinal therapies. It is also found in some shampoos.

Common uses include:

• Arthritis

Nutmeg

This spice is best known for its culinary uses, especially in desserts and fruit dishes. However, both nutmeg powder and the essential oil have medicinal properties.

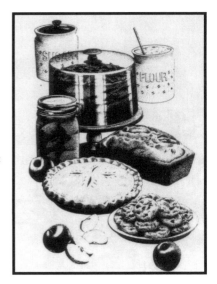

Common uses include:

• Acne
• Insomnia

Oatstraw

This herb is rich in many vitamins and minerals, and it is also a source of fiber. It has antiseptic and other medicinal qualities.

Common uses include:

• Prostate problems

Oregano

Oregano is closely related to marjoram, and like that herb, is best known for its role in the kitchen. It is found extensively in Italian and other Mediterranean cuisines. However, it does have some medical applications as well.

Common uses include:

- Bruises
- Colds
- Coughs
- Indigestion
- Sinusitis

Parsley

This plant is commonly found in herb gardens, much prized for its culinary properties. It was held in high regard by the ancient Greeks, who used it in their funeral rites. In cooking, it adds flavor to soups, sauces, stuffings, salads, and many other dishes. Medicinally, an infusion of parsley has traditionally been used to treat various ailments.

Common uses include:

- Arthritis
- Bad breath
- Body odor
- Bruises
- Colds
- Diabetes
- Edema
- Eye problems
- Flatulence
- Flu
- Gall bladder problems
- Hemorrhoids
- High blood pressure
- Menstrual problems
- PMS

Passionflower

This plant produces colorful flowers, and some varieties yield edible fruit. It has long been of great service in homeopathic medicine.

Common uses include:

- Insomnia
- Nervousness
- Stress

Pau d'arco

The bark from this Brazilian tree has long been valued throughout South America for its healing powers. It was one of the primary medicinal herbs of the ancient Incas and Aztecs. It appears to have antibacterial, antiviral, and antifungal properties.

Common uses include:

• Inflammation   • Nervousness   • Stress

Peppermint

This herb has many culinary uses. It is widely used as a flavoring, particularly in candy. A soothing, flavorful tea can be brewed from its leaves. Additionally, it has medical applications, usually as an infusion of its leaves or using the essential oil.

Common uses include:

• Bad breath   • Dandruff   • Heartburn
• Body odor   • Fatigue (aromatherapy)   • Impotence
• Breastfeeding   • Flatulence   • Indigestion
• Colic   • Gall bladder problems   • Motion sickness
• Coughs   • Headaches   • Nausea

Pipsissewa

Also known as the Prince's Pine, this evergreen can be found on four continents—Europe, Asia, and the Americas. Its leaves have a variety of medicinal properties.

Common uses include:

• Bladder infections   • Kidney problems

Raspberry Leaves

The raspberry grows wild in many areas and is cultivated for its delicious fruit. An infusion made from its leaves has long been a remedy prescribed by traditional healers.

Common uses include:

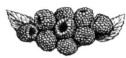

- Diarrhea
- High blood pressure
- Leg cramps
- PMS
- Weight control

Red Clover

These plants grow wild in meadows. They are valued by herbalists for their flowerheads, which are dried before using. Red clover is an expectorant and contains other medicinal properties as well.

Common uses include:

- Hay fever
- Inflammation

Rose

These flowers are both beautiful and versatile. Rose hips, usually taken in the form of a tea, are highly nutritious and are an especially rich source of vitamin C. Roses are also used in the production of some candies and of course perfumes. Medicinally, rose leaves have astringent and laxative properties. The essential oil from the variety rosa gallica is used in aromatherapy.

Common uses include:

- Arthritis
- Constipation (aromatherapy)

Rosemary

This shrubby plant is a favorite of many herb gardens. Its evergreen leaves have a pleasant, pungent scent. Much symbolic lore is attached to the herb. According to ancient folk wisdom, it strengthens the memory. Historically, it has held an important place in various religious rituals and festivals, including both weddings and funerals. Medieval brides wore wreaths of rosemary. The herb has various medicinal properties, and oil of rosemary is used in aromatherapy.

Common uses include:

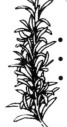

- Arthritis
- Eye problems
- Fatigue (aromatherapy)

- Headache
- Memory problems (aromatherapy)
- Stress (aromatherapy)

Sacred Bark

This herb is also commonly referred to as cascara sagada. It is well-known for its laxative properties and was used by Native American healers.

Common uses include:

- Constipation

Sage

This aromatic herb is widely used in cooking, most notably in the stuffing for Thanksgiving turkey. Native Americans burned sage to cleanse and purify sacred places. For centuries, it has been highly regarded for its healing powers and has been used to treat a variety of ailments. It is usually taken as an infusion, however the oil of certain varieties of sage is also used in aromatherapy.

• Herbs & Their Uses •

Common uses include:

- Arthritis
- Bad breath
- Body odor
- Diabetes
- Frostbite
- Hair loss
- Indigestion
- Insomnia
- Memory problems
- Nervousness
- Stress
- Toothache

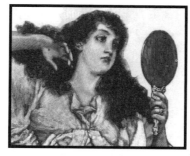

Sandalwood

This small tree, native to India, is highly prized for its oil and wood. Sandalwood oil has a rich, luxurious scent and is widely used in perfume and bath oils. It has medical properties as well. The wood is often used to make decorative, carved objects.

Common uses include:

- Hiccups (aromatherapy)
- Stress (aromatherapy)
- Nervousness (aromatherapy)

Savory

This flowering plant with its hot, peppery flavor is used primarily as a culinary herb, to add zest to vegetable, bean, and meat dishes. It was first utilized by the Romans in their cooking. It has some medicinal uses.

Common uses include:

- Aphrodisiac

Saw Palmetto

This plant is a small palm tree that is native to the east coast of the United States. It is an effective expectorant and has many other medicinal applications as well.

Common uses include:

- Frigidity
- Prostate problems

Senna

This herb comes from a small shrub and yields a powerful medicine that has long been employed by traditional healers, as far back as the ancient Greeks. It is most noted for its laxative properties.

Common uses include:

- Constipation

Sesame

These seeds are highly nutritious, a rich source of vitamins and minerals. They are used in baking, and the seeds and oil extracted from them are used extensively in Middle Eastern cuisine. The oil has a number of medicinal applications.

Common uses include:

- Arthritis
- Ears ringing
- Ear wax buildup
- Frigidity
- Sore muscles
- Stress

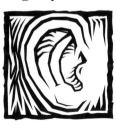

Slippery Elm

This small tree grows prolifically in various parts of North America. There are no applications for its wood, but the bark is highly prized by traditional healers. Slippery elm bark was much utilized by Native Americans. Today, this herb is sold mostly in powdered form. It is highly nutritious and has a soothing, healing effect.

Common uses include:

- Colds
- Coughs
- Heartburn
- Indigestion
- Smoking

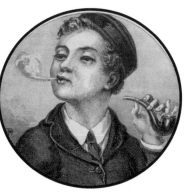

Squaw Vine

This herb is exclusively American in origin and was used by Native American healers. As the name indicates, it was mostly taken by Native American women, just before childbirth to make it safer and easier.

Common uses include:

- Menstrual problems
- PMS

Stone Root

This plant, native to North America, grows mostly in moist and wooded environments. As its name suggests, it is valued for its root. Herbalists have long used it for a variety of medicinal purposes.

Common uses include:

- Hemorrhoids

287

Suma

This herb was first utilized by tribes of indigenous peoples in Brazil. It is sometimes referred to as the "South American ginseng." It is used as a tonic for overall healthfulness and is reputed to help correct hormonal imbalances in women.

Common uses include:

- Menopause
- Menstrual problems
- PMS

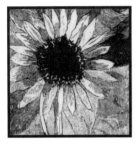

Sunflower

These tall plants are actually weeds, but are planted for their cheerful flowers and their seeds. The seeds are highly nutritious and have a variety of medicinal applications as well.

Common uses include:

- Asthma
- Colds
- Constipation
- Coughs
- Eye problems
- High cholesterol
- Memory problems
- Smoking

Thyme

This herb is popular in the kitchen, and is often used to spice up meat and poultry dishes, as well as soups and stuffings. It has a wide array of medicinal applications. Extracts of the herb are contained in some commercial mouthwashes and liniments.

Common uses include:

- Dandruff

Uva Ursi

This plant grows indigenously in Europe, Asia, and the Americas. Its Latin name means "the bear's grape," and it is also commonly referred to as bearberry. Uva ursi is a diuretic and was used extensively in Medieval medicine.

Common uses include:

- Bladder infections
- Incontinence
- Kidney problems

Valerian

This plant is valued for its root and produces a powerful medicine. It is well-known for its sedative effect, among other medicinal properties.

Common uses include:

- Back pain
- Hyperactivity
- Insomnia
- Nervousness
- Stress

Watermelon Seed

In addition to being a refreshing and delicious summertime fruit, watermelon has medicinal applications when its seeds are ground and made into a tea.

Common uses include:

- Bladder infections
- High blood pressure
- Kidney problems
- Water retention

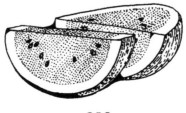

Wheatgrass

Often taken as a natural food supplement, wheatgrass is rich in a variety of vitamins, minerals and trace elements. It has some therapeutic value as well.

Common uses include:

• Bad breath   • Body Odor

White Oak

The bark of this tree is highly astringent and is used by herbalists to treat a number of maladies. It can be taken both internally and externally.

Common uses include:

• Poison Ivy and Poison Oak   • Snakebite

White Willow

This tree grows throughout the United States in moist environments, usually alongside rivers and streams. Medicinally, it is prized for its bark that contains the same active ingredient as aspirin. Like the over-the-counter medication, it effectively relieves pain and reduces fevers.

Common uses include:

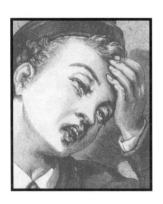

• Back pain   • Infections
• Fever   • Sore muscles
• Headache

Wild Yam

The root of this plant has many medicinal applications. In Southern China, certain varieties are used to produce dyes.

Common uses include:

- Gallbladder Problems

Wormwood

The herb takes its official name, artemisia absinthium, from the Greek goddess Artemis who was associated with women in childbirth. During ancient times, it was a favorite remedy for female complaints. Its common name comes from its use in getting rid of worms. The herb has an extremely bitter taste and was used to flavor absinthe, an alcoholic beverage produced in France that has long since been banned because of the long-term damage it does to the nervous system. Today, wormwood still has a few medicinal applications.

Common uses include:

- Worms

Yarrow

This common herb grows just about everywhere, in meadows, ditches, and alongside roads. It derives its Latin name, achillea millefolium, from the ancient story that Achilles used it to treat his soldiers' wounds. Yarrow has a wide variety of medicinal and occasional culinary uses.

Common uses include:

• Back Pain	• Flu	• Nausea
• Cuts and Scrapes	• Gout	• Oily Skin
• Diabetes	• Menstrual Problems	• Toothache

Yellow Dock

This plant grows wild as a weed and is classified in the same family as rhubarb. Its root is used medicinally. Herbalists value it primarily for its gentle laxative action, but it has a few additional medicinal applications as well.

Common uses include:

• Psoriasis

Yerba Mate

This is a caffeinated tea-like beverage, made from the herb yerba, that is popular in many parts of South America. It is greenish in color and is valued for its stimulating effect. It is nutritious, containing several vitamins and minerals.

Common uses include:

• Memory Problems   • Weight Control

Yucca root

Yucca is a desert plant that produces edible fruit. Its root has a variety of medicinal uses and may act as a laxative.

Common uses include:

• Arthritis

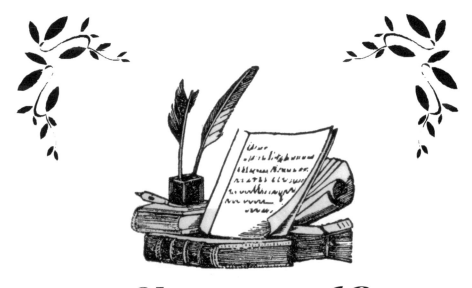

Chapter 18

GLOSSARY OF TERMS

Acidophilus -
lactobacillus acidophilus. A "friendly" form of bacteria that lives in the human gastrointestinal tract and aids in digestion. It is found in yogurt with active cultures. There are also supplements in various forms currently on the market.

Activated Charcoal -
a form of carbon, high porous, that easily absorbs other materials. It is used in emergency rooms to treat certain kinds of poisoning and has many useful applications in home healing.

Acupressure -
a traditional therapy in Asian medicine that involves applying manual pressure to parts of the body to relieve various symptoms and treat illnesses.

• Glossary Of Terms •

Aerobic -
in the presence of oxygen. Aerobic exercise conditions the heart and lungs and increases the body's efficiency of oxygen intake.

Allicin -
a yellowish, oily liquid extracted from garlic that has anti-bacterial properties.

Alum -
an astringent substance used in the manufacture of baking powder, dyes, and other materials. It is one of the key ingredients in the pickling process.

Amino acid -
the chemical compound that forms the building blocks of protein. There are twenty-five different amino acids.

Analgesic -
a class of drugs that are used to reduce pain.

Antabuse -
a drug used in the treatment of alcoholism that makes ingesting alcohol physically unpleasant.

Antihistamine -
a drug that counteracts allergic reactions.

Aromatherapy -
a therapy using various scents, from the essential oils of plants, to strengthen physical and emotional well-being. It is one of several therapies used in alternative healing.

Bile -
a bitter fluid produced by the liver and stored in the gall bladder that aids in digestion.

• *Glossary Of Terms* •

Bilirubin -
a yellowish-red pigment found in bile.

Bonemeal -
a compound of finely ground bones that are used to feed stock animals, as fertilizer, and as a nutritional supplement for humans.

Brewer's Yeast -
also called nutritional yeast. It is rich in many basic nutrients, including B-complex and other vitamins, amino acids, and numerous minerals, and is therefore often taken as a natural food supplement.

Bronchi -
the two major branches of the trachea that lead into the lungs.

Bronchioles -
smaller sub-sections of the bronchi.

Capsaicin -
a substance found in hot peppers that has a burning taste. It has numerous medicinal applications.

Carbohydrate -
an organic substance that provides energy to the body, including sugars, starch, and cellulose.

Chlorophyll -
a green pigment found in plant cells that is essential to photosynthesis, the process by which plants create the nutritional matter they need.

Cholesterol -
a chemical found in foods, often those high in fat. A small amount of cholesterol is necessary for the body's normal functioning; an excessive amount can be dangerous, leading to narrowing of the blood vessels and increased risk of stroke and heart disease.

• Glossary Of Terms •

Conjunctivitis -
an inflammation of the transparent membrane that lines the eyelid and outer eye. It is also known as "pink eye" since the eye is usually noticeably red and irritated.

Diuretic -
a substance that tends to increase the urine flow or leads to the excretion of fluids.

Eczema -
a specific form of dermatitis or skin inflammation that is usually caused by an allergic reaction.

Edema -
retention of fluids in tissues that leads to swelling.

Epsom Salts -
a chemical compound rich in magnesium that is often used in therapeutic baths and footsoaks. It has long been valued for its healing properties.

Escherichia Coli -
a form of bacteria that is commonly found in the human digestive tract.

Essential Oil -
any volatile oil that gives a distinctive taste or scent to a plant, flower, or fruit. These oils are used extensively in aromatherapy.

Estrogen -
female sex hormone.

Furuncle -
another term for a boil.

Gamma Linolenic Acid (GLA) -
a substance that is synthesized in the body from essential fatty acids. GLA has numerous functions in various bodily systems.

Herpes Simplex -
a virus in humans that produces cold sores.

Hypothalamus -
the portion of the brain that regulates many aspects of metabolism, including body temperature.

Kidney stones -
accumulations of mineral salts (mostly combined with calcium) which can lodge along the urinary tract. Symptoms of kidney stones include pain radiating from the lower abdomen to the upper back, frequent urination with blood and pus in the urine, and sometimes fever and chills.

L-lysine -
an amino acid that is an essential building block of all protein.

Larynx -
the upper part of the trachea. Contains the vocal chords.

Lactose -
a type of sugar that is present in milk and milk products.

Lactose intolerance -
a condition in which one lacks the enzyme to digest lactose. As a result, eating milk products (except for yogurt and certain cheeses) produces a lot of gas and may cause diarrhea.

Lecithin -
a nutrient needed by every cell in the body. Cell membranes are largely made up of lecithin, and without this nutrient, they would

harden. Lecithin can be made in the body, although lecithin supplements, made mostly from soybeans, are available in granules, capsules and liquid form.

Legumes -
the fruit or seed of certain plants used for food. Beans, some peas and nuts fall into this category.

Linoleic Acid -
a liquid, unsaturated fatty acid, that is found in most vegetables and vegetable oils (except coconut or palm kernel oil). It is the most essential fatty acid.

Lyme Disease -
a disease carried by the tiny deer tick. It takes its name from the town of Lyme, Connecticut, where it was first discovered. Lyme disease is a serious condition which should be treated as soon as the tick bite is discovered, or the symptoms occur. These include a rash, flu-like symptoms, fatigue, headache, stiff neck, backache, nausea and vomiting.

Malaria -
a disease caused by parasites in red blood cells. It is transmitted by the bite of certain mosquitoes. It is characterized by periodic bouts of chills and fever.

Metabolism -
the process by which energy is provided for vital bodily processes and activities through the assimilation of new materials.

Ovulation -
the part of the menstrual cycle when an egg is released from the ovary.

Oxidation -
a chemical reaction that occurs when oxygen is added, producing a chemical transformation.

• Glossary Of Terms •

Parotid glands -
the pair of large glands situated below and in front of the ears.

Pectin -
a water-soluble substance that binds with adjacent cells to form a gel. It is found in some fruits and vegetables including apples, carrots, citrus fruits, beets, bananas and cabbage and is the basis for fruit jellies.

Peristalsis -
the involuntary wave-like contractions that force food along the esophagus and the intestines.

Psyllium Seed -
one of the most popular fibers, psyllium seed is a good intestinal cleanser and stool softener. Some of the over-the-counter laxative formulas contain this natural fiber supplement.

Quinine -
a bitter crystalline alkaloid extracted from sinchona bark that is used in medicine for a variety of purposes—especially in the treatment of malaria.

Resin -
organic substances excreted from plants and trees.

Ringworm -
any of several contagious fungal diseases that affect the skin, hair and nails of humans and domestic animals.

Rocky Mountain Spotted Fever -
an acute disease transmitted by a tick—especially the American dog tick or a wood tick. Symptoms include fever, chills, muscle and joint pains.

Salmonella -
a bacteria that can cause among other things, food poisoning and gastrointestinal inflammation.

· Glossary Of Terms ·

Sitz bath -
a form of hydrotherapy, this is a therapeutic bath taken in a sitting position. Epsom salts and certain medicinal herbs are often added to the bathwater.

Solanine-
a bitter, poisonous crystalline compound from several plants belonging to the nightshade family.

Thrush -
a fungal infection that occurs most often in infants. It is characterized by white spots in the mouth.

Trachea -
the windpipe.

Tryptophan -
an essential amino acid, widely distributed in proteins. It is known to create drowsiness in humans.

Uric acid -
an acid that is present in urine.

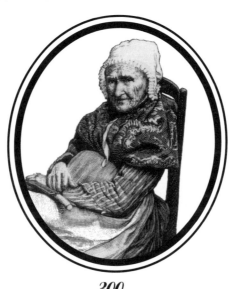

C

E

· Index ·

Eggplant, 35, 107, 189
Eggs, 20, 34; hard-boiled, 53; shells of, 102; whites of, 11, 35-36, 46, 51, 57, 151, 207
Elderberry, 268; blue syrup, 68; black syrup, 68; juice, 60
Enemas, 138-139, 159
Escarole, 140
Espom salts, 18, 27, 110, 115, 129-130, 251, 296, 300
Eucalyptus, 61, 268; oil, 17, 55-57, 60, 111, 164, 175
Eucerin, 33
Exercise, 58, 107, 118, 129, 139, 150, 178, 186, 190, 192, 196, 233-234, 237, 241-242, 244, 252, 294
Expectorants, 57, 258, 277, 283, 286
Eyebright, 79, 268; tea, 248
Eyes, 120, 296; bloodshot, 4, 79, 274; burning, 79; irritated, 4, 79, 81-82, 170; problems with, 4, 79, 263, 268-269, 271, 281, 284, 288; puffy, 4, 83-84; sensitivity to light, 79; tired, 4, 81-82
Eyesight, 4, 80-81. See also Eyes.
Eyestrain, 4, 81. See also Eyes.

F

Facial masks, 3, 12, 34-37. See also Skin.
Fat, 10, 50, 61, 89, 145, 187, 196, 241; bacon, 21; beef, 21
Fatigue, 8, 198-199, 234, 237, 240-241, 271, 273, 276, 282, 284, 298
Fels-Naptha soap, 10, 43
Fennel, 197, 208, 229, 268, 278; dried, 226; seeds, 68, 82, 148, 204; tea, 70, 82, 148, 155, 226
Fenugreek, 269; seed, 77; tea, 65, 77, 169, 211
Feverfew, 127, 269
Fevers, 4, 56, 66-67, 120, 167, 277, 278, 290, 298-299
Fiber, 15, 137-138, 141, 144, 183, 189, 196, 299
Figs, 19, 52, 142
Fish, 110, 187, 205; liver oil, 238; oil, 109
Fissures, 5, 148
Flatulence, 5, 148-150, 205, 208, 210, 256-257, 263-264, 269-271, 276, 281-282, 297
Flaxseeds, 115, 138, 140, 202, 269; ground, 39; oil of, 39, 184
Flour, 20; white, 126
Flus, 4, 54-55, 68-69, 262, 264, 267, 269, 271, 281, 291

Fo ti, 229, 270
Food poisoning, 7, 205-206, 271, 299
Frigidity, 8, 229-230, 259, 266, 270-271, 277, 286
Frostbite, 7, 183-184, 271, 274, 285
Fructose, 158
Fruits, 88, 138, 158, 189, 195, 219, 238, 241, 299; citrus, 206; dried, 39; juices of, 189, 221; raw, 200
Fungal infections, 6, 16, 58, 158, 174, 270. See also Infections.
Furuncle. See Boils.

G

Gall bladders, 294; problems of, 7, 197-198, 258, 262, 267, 269, 281-282, 291
Gargles, 70-71, 73, 135
Garlic, 16, 19, 34, 53, 56, 58, 64, 73, 93, 103, 113, 120, 143, 151, 158, 166-167, 183, 185, 189, 196, 200, 202, 231, 270, 294; dried, 58; enemas, 159; juice, 122; oil, 73, 76; pickled, 200; pills, 113, 176, 231, 238; raw, 48
Gin, 57, 236, 275
Ginger, 31, 56, 60, 64, 79, 81, 129, 174, 183-184, 206, 215, 218, 245, 270; capsules, 213, 215-216; juice, 111, 130; powdered, 56, 59, 215; tea, 68, 144, 149, 165, 206, 235
Ginger ale, 71, 204, 216
Gingko biloba, 127, 242, 271; capsules, 252
Ginseng, 229, 231, 233, 242, 271; Korean, 15, 196; Siberian, 163
Goldenseal, 32, 43, 45, 79, 141, 159, 174; powder, 102; tea, 55, 120, 189, 199
Gooseberries, 68-69
Gota kola, 15, 231-233, 248, 252
Gout, 5, 119-120, 265, 267, 270, 274-275, 291
Grains, whole, 40, 125, 138, 157, 195, 204, 219, 234, 241
Grapefruits, 130, 140, 189, 222; juice of, 56, 142, 157, 197; peels of, 211
Grapes, 67; juice of, 67, 156; vine leaves of, 151; white juice of, 110
Green tea, 69
Guarana, 242, 273
Gums, bleeding, 4, 89. See also Mouth.

H

Hair, 299; loss, 8, 230, 285
Hangovers, 8, 221-223

304

· Index ·

S

Sacred bark, 141, 284

Sage, 112, 246, 284; tea, 97, 183, 197, 211, 226, 230, 248, 250

Salacin, 117

Salmon oil, 107

Salt, 16-17, 20, 30, 49, 52, 88, 96, 108, 141, 147, 170, 175, 182, 184, 186, 201, 206, 210, 234, 236, 244; sea, 68, 70; table, 74; water, 38, 90, 95

Salves, 94, 111, 118

Sandalwood, 285; oil, 172

Sauerkraut, 25; juice, 55, 141, 145

Savory, 285

Saw palmetto, 229, 239, 286

Scars, 14, 26

Scrapes, 5, 101-102, 262, 291

Seafood, 163

Seaweed, 113, 251, 276

Senility, 8, 252, 257, 260

Senna, 141, 286

Sesame, 286; oil, 78, 111, 130; seeds, 230, 251

Shiitake mushrooms. See Mushrooms.

Shingles, 6, 160-161, 256

Shortness of breath, 6, 175. See also Breath.

Showers, 37-38, 66, 78, 213, 242

Silver dollar, 85

Sinus, 68, 73, 75, 120, 123, 177; problems, 170. See also Sinusitis.

Sinusitis, 6, 175-177, 268, 270, 274, 281

Skin, 9-53, 158, 160, 299; cancer, 3, 48; dry, 3, 9-10, 14, 33-34; itchy, 3, 29, 37-39, 42-47, 150, 161, 264, 269; leathery, 37; oily, 3, 10, 35, 41-42, 263, 277, 291; problems, 12, 160, 263, 270, 276

Slippery elm bark, 57, 206, 208, 287; powder, 57, 206, 223; tea, 61, 206, 224

Smoking, 8, 34, 76, 79, 86, 175, 223-224, 264-265, 270, 278, 287-288

Snakebites, 5, 104, 265, 290. See also Bites.

Snoring, 6, 177-179

Soaps, 42, 99, 226-227, 276

Solanine, 107, 300

Sore throats, 4, 56, 65, 69-73, 158, 262-263, 265, 270-271, 274, 277, 279, 286

Sores: bed, 3, 19, 270; canker, 4, 89-92, 158, 279; cold, 4, 92-95, 183, 256, 261, 265, 270, 279, 297. See also Mouth.

Soup, 199-200; chicken, 56

Sour cream, 49, 144

Soybeans, 190, 199, 298; black, 139

Spinach, 19, 140, 280

Splinters, 5, 104

Squaw: bush, 235; vine, 237, 287

Strawberries, 12, 120, 123, 251

Stone root, 151, 287

Stress, 8, 19, 45, 120, 184, 215, 229, 243, 252-253, 263-264, 273, 276, 281-282, 284-286, 289

String beans. See Beans.

Strokes, 188, 295

Stys, 4, 83. See also Eyes.

Sugar, 23, 66, 126, 143, 148, 156, 158, 171, 195, 196, 237, 241-242, 297; brown, 62, 205; cube, 164; high intake of, 79, 92

Sulfites, 163

Sulfur, 34

Summa, 288; capsules, 233, 236; tea, 185

Sunburn, 3, 47, 49-51, 256

Sunflower, 288; seeds, 57, 65, 81, 143, 165-166, 188, 224, 247, 288

Sunlight, 14, 30, 46, 93

Sunscreen, 14, 93

T

Tapeworm, 5, 104-105. See also Fungal infections.

Tartar, cream of, 130, 213

Tea, 11, 21-22, 28, 31, 35, 42-43, 45, 48-49, 55-56, 59, 60-61, 64-68, 70-73, 77, 80, 82, 97, 104, 112, 115, 119-120, 124, 127, 129, 134, 136, 144-145, 147-149, 155-156, 159-160, 169-170, 174, 176, 183, 187, 189, 191, 197-199, 201-202, 204, 206, 208, 211-212, 214-215, 217-218, 223-224, 226, 229-231, 235-239, 245-246, 248, 250, 252, 280, 282; bags, 21, 28, 51, 53, 73, 82-83, 91, 102

Tea tree oil, 17

Thyme, 31, 288; oil, 31

Tobacco, 100-101

Tofu, 44

Tomato, 107; juice, 156, 220; products, 206

Toothaches, 4, 96-98, 256, 262-263, 265, 285, 291. See also Mouth.

Touch-me-nots. See Jewelweed.

Toxins, 21, 56, 59, 104, 108, 110, 119, 220, 226, 255

Turnips, 23, 62, 189; juice of, 227

· *Index* ·

U

Ulcers, 7, 217-218, 256, 258, 262-263, 271, 277; leg, 160
Under-eye puffiness, 4, 83-84. See also Eyes.
Uric acid, 119, 300
Urine, 11, 119,133, 200-201, 297, 300
Uva ursi, 289; capsules, 136; tea, 134

V

Valerian root, 115, 246, 289; capsules, 243, 252; extract, 243
Vanilla extract, 25-26, 97
Vaporizers, 164, 175
Varicose veins, 7, 190-193, 257-258, 261
Vaseline, 33, 58, 148, 160
Vegetables, 126, 138, 157, 195, 209, 219, 241, 261, 298-299; leafy green, 39, 88, 125, 181, 190, 204, 234, 237-238; juices of, 189, 239; oils, 36, 130, 181; raw, 137, 200; steamed, 137
Vick's Vapor Rub, 123, 177
Vinegar, 12, 26-28, 85, 121, 158, 166; apple cider, 12, 16, 30, 41, 49, 63, 70-71, 94, 110, 123, 126, 131, 145, 169, 171, 191, 193, 198, 207, 212, 227, 240; white, 18, 29, 67; white cider, 12
Viruses, 51, 54, 58, 68, 89, 92, 159, 174-175
Vision, blurred, 4, 79-80, 256. See also Eyes.
Vitamin A, 117, 238, 259, 261, 268
Vitamin B, 92-93, 145, 154, 247, 268
Vitamin B-1, 259
Vitamin B-2, 79, 259
Vitamin B-6, 108, 125, 195, 201, 216, 237, 243
Vitamin B-12, 247
Vitamin C, 22, 68, 92-93, 108, 124, 137, 150, 166, 168, 221, 259, 261, 266, 268, 280, 283
Vitamin D, 107, 117, 259
Vitamin E, 14, 32, 102, 108, 125, 168, 181, 188, 191, 232; capsules, 50, 161; oil, 26, 28, 94, 152, 259
Vitamin K, 191, 266
Vodka, 77, 87

W

Walnuts, ground, 94
Warts, 3, 51-53, 267, 270; plantar, 52
Water retention, 6, 155, 289
Watercress, 196
Watermelon: rind, 47; seed, 185, 201, 289; tea, 155

Weight control, 6, 155-156, 196, 265, 269, 273, 283, 292
Wheat: germ, 140; oil, 152; products, 158
Wheatgrass, 227, 290
Whiskey, 59, 63, 97. See also Liquor.
White oat bark, 104, 290; tea, 42
White willow bark, 117, 290; powdered, 116
Whooping cough, 6, 179, See also Coughs.
Wild yam, 197, 291
Wine: dry red, 63; mulled, 63; red, 95; white, 57, 184
Wintergreen oil, 116
Witch hazel, 22, 38, 124, 151-152, 175, 184, 193
Worms, 5, 105, 263, 291
Wormwood, 105, 291
Wrinkles, 3, 34-36, 50, 53, 265

Y

Yarrow, 101-102, 115, 291; dried, 42; tea, 42, 68, 98, 119, 197, 215, 236
Yeast, 47, 158; brewer's, 79, 93, 103, 140, 154, 169, 188, 195, 234, 295
Yellow dock, 45, 292
Yerba mate tea, 155, 248, 292
Yogurt, 30, 35, 49, 91, 93, 137, 144, 149, 158, 293
Yucca root, 109, 292

Z

Zinc, 10, 14, 66, 108, 226; lozenges, 72; oxide, 152
Zucchini, 209

309